D1155997

Making Sense of Psychiatric Cases

MAURICE GREENBERG
Consultant Psychiatrist and Honorary Senior Lecturer,
University College Hospital and Student Health Centre,
University College, London

GEORGE SZMUKLER
Senior Lecturer in Psychiatry, Institute of Psychiatry;
Honorary Consultant Psychiatrist, Bethlem Royal and Maudsley
Hospital

DIGBY TANTAM
Senior Lecturer in Psychiatry, Victoria University of
Manchester; Honorary Consultant Psychiatrist, University
Hospital of South Manchester

OXFORD   NEW YORK   TOKYO
OXFORD UNIVERSITY PRESS
1986

Oxford University Press, Walton Street, Oxford OX2 6DP

Oxford New York Toronto
Delhi Bombay Calcutta Madras Karachi
Kuala Lumpur Singapore Hong Kong Tokyo
Nairobi Dar es Salaam Cape Town
Melbourne Auckland

and associated companies in
Beirut Berlin Ibadan Nicosia

Oxford is a trade mark of Oxford University Press

British Library Cataloguing in Publication Data
Greenberg, Maurice
Making sense of psychiatric cases.
1. Psychiatry—Case studies
I. Title   II. Szmukler, George   III. Tantam,
Digby
616.89′09   RC465
ISBN 0-19-261437-1

Library of Congress Cataloging in Publication Data
Greenberg, Maurice.
Making sense of psychiatric cases.
(Oxford medical publications)
Includes index.
1. Psychiatry—Case studies. 2. Mental illness—
Diagnosis—Case studies. 3. Psychotherapy—Case
studies. I. Szmukler, George. II. Tantam, Digby.
III. Title. IV. Series. [DNLM: 1. Mental Disorders—
case studies. 2. Psychiatry—methods. WM 40 G789m]
RC465.G744   1986   616.89′09   85-15398
ISBN 0-19-261437-1 (pbk.)

Set by Cotswold Typesetting, Cheltenham
Printed in Great Britain
at the University Press, Oxford
by David Stanford
Printer to the University

Foreword

Gerald Russell *Professor of Psychiatry, Institute of Psychiatry and the Maudsley Hospital, London*

Mentally ill patients are always more interesting than psychiatrists' accounts of their disorders. This is hardly surprising as nothing can surpass the immediacy of hearing the patient tell us about his inner chaos and distress. Nevertheless many psychiatric texts suffer unnecessarily from their authors' eagerness to simplify and explain. Apart from losing sight of the humanity of the patients' stories they run risks by taking short cuts through the entanglements of clinical psychiatry. Drs Greenberg, Szmukler, and Tantam have written this book so as to present a method of collecting and ordering clinical facts, with a view to doing justice to the patient's needs. They provide serialized case-histories and invite the reader to follow successive episodes, thus piecing together the jig-saw that will lead to the diagnosis, an elucidation of likely causes, and a plan of management tailored to the individual patient. It is precisely because this book's clinical case histories ring true in their complexity that the reader's interest will be captured. He should be carried from one episode to the next as the story unfolds, and learn how to utilize fresh data gathered through the clinician's enquiries or yielded in response to his therapeutic endeavours.

From this book the newcomer to psychiatry can learn how to develop skills in the most vital and basic procedures of clinical practice. He might also be spared some of the painful steps of trial and error, from which the acquisition of clinical experience is not entirely divorced. The method described leads logically to a multi-dimensional view of causation and an eclectic approach to treatment. If he remembers these lessons, the reader should avoid a mechanistic type of practice whereby treatment is ordered merely in response to a diagnosis with insufficient regard for the patient's personal needs.

The authors of this book deserve praise for their originality and enterprise. The book is original because it describes sound

clinical methods not readily available save by serving an appren-
ticeship in a good teaching centre. The enterprise is evident from
the authors' willingness to express their views without seeking
refuge behind citations from standard texts. The reader is
advised to consult this book in a receptive frame of mind, and
not assume prematurely that he already knows the best
approaches to psychiatric practice. Even the experienced
psychiatrist will encounter fresh food for thought in this lively
and enjoyable book.

Preface

This book is about psychological problems as they appear in clinical practice. Our goal is to show how information obtained from the patient and others can be built up into a form which is most useful for researching a psychiatric diagnosis and deciding on management. The process of 'formulating' a case is frequently complex, yet we believe that it constitutes a key skill in psychiatry. Management cannot be based on diagnosis alone, or indeed on any other single characteristic, but requires the appraisal of, amongst other things, relevant aspects of the patient's personality, experience, and social context. Which of these is important will vary from patient to patient but will be contained in a useful formulation of that patient's problem. The formulation holds within itself the complexity of a case but at the same time offers a prescription for action.

Although this book was written with psychiatric trainees, senior medical students, and general practitioners in mind, we hope it will also prove helpful for other professionals who feel in need of some guidance in approaching patients with psychological problems. This is because it deals with how psychiatric knowledge is applied to particular cases, a skill separate from the acquisition of such knowledge. However, it has been assumed that the reader already knows something about psychiatry and this book is intended to complement, but not replace, talking with patients and studying relevant literature.

Our experience has been that the best way to teach medical students how to formulate a case is to confront them with a real situation. The same practice has been followed in this book where cases have been chosen to illustrate common and important clinical problems. These cases are not 'idealized' as this would have made them less convincing, but they are disguised in order to conceal the identities of the patients. Because our intention is to show readers how we think about what we do, and we hope that they will make their own judgements, there are likely to be disagreements over some of the cases we describe. We welcome this, provided that support for alternative views can be

vii

marshalled from the case material. Such disagreements are inevitable if the reality of clinical situations is to be reflected.

Readers are encouraged to approach this book in an active manner. The cases have therefore been presented in a format which provides appropriate breaks where we ask readers to develop their own formulations before moving on to ours.

We suggest that the reader starts with the first chapter because this introduces the structure we use and shows how historical details collected from a number of sources and not presented in any sort of order can be integrated into a coherent and psychiatrically useful narrative. The second chapter illustrates the value of actively pursuing a fresh enquiry at different times in a patient's history. This and subsequent chapters are, however, self-contained and can be read in any order.

Each of the case studies begins with an account of the history and examination organized along the lines presented in Chapter 1. An initial formulation is added to or changed in the light of further information obtained, with the search for this information being guided by the earlier formulation. There is no 'final' formulation because this would imply that all the questions about a particular case have been answered and the matter closed. This, in our experience, is a state of affairs rarely encountered.

M.G.

London and Manchester   G.S.

D.T.

Acknowledgements

Many people have read and commented on parts of this book. In particular, we would like to thank Dr Peter Noble who generously undertook the task of reading the manuscript, and the consultants who gave their permission for us to use their cases. Their advice has been invaluable in helping us to clarify our ideas, but we remain ultimately responsible for the finished product.

We also wish to thank Maggy Gleeson, Mary Haywood, and Lilian Gaywood who typed the manuscript.

To our wives,
Marion, Linnet, and Sheila

Contents

1

How to organize and select information—the case of Mr Daniels, aged 17

Presenting complaint

The staff of a local day centre contacted the hospital to ask for help. Mr Daniels, a 17-year-old Guyanese-born man who had been attending the day centre regularly for some time, had recently begun to behave strangely and they felt that they could no longer cope with him. The last straw was when he came into a staff meeting, insisting that he was a member of staff, and spent the meeting kneeling in a position of prayer, making bellowing noises.

On further questioning over the telephone the member of staff added that Mr Daniels had been behaving strangely for several days, and that he had stated on different occasions that he was dead and that half his brain was linked to the moon. It was thought that he would probably need admission, and it was suggested that he be brought immediately to the hospital.

When he arrived Mr Daniels sat down in the examining psychiatrist's room but kept his eyes closed and either refused to answer questions or shouted 'no' to them. He would, however, respond to simple requests and it was possible to make a superficial physical examination which showed an axillary temperature of 38.5°C and a radial pulse rate of 120 per minute. He seemed hostile and suspicious but not depressed.

At this point, Mr Daniel's mother, who worked nearby, arrived. She said that Mr Daniels appeared well until two weeks before, when he visited her and seemed rather restless. A week before, on another visit, he had sworn at her, 'a sure sign of illness' according to his mother, and tried to set fire to a book on the kitchen stove, saying, 'after this I'll be all right because I'll be thinking straight'. During this visit, he had an argument with his

1

father and he told the family that he thought that he should go to the hospital but his father told him not to, saying it was for 'fools'. Mr Daniels then picked up a kitchen knife and stood with it behind the kitchen door. The family disarmed him and his father banned him from the parental home, refusing to accept his wife's explanation that their son was ill. Two days before admission, the parents came home to find their front door broken down, the furniture smashed or disarranged, and their son emptying the kitchen cupboards.

Mrs Daniels could give no other information, saying that she only saw her son occasionally, when he visited. She had not, however, thought her son's mood was more depressed than usual, nor had she noted any weight loss. She did report that her son had had a previous admission, and the notes were sent for.

The discharge letter to the general practitioner stated that the previous admission had followed a three-month illness characterized by religiosity, aggressiveness (he had tried to strangle his sister), the belief that he was a person with special powers and the perception of a smell of rotten pork emanating from other people. He had had a pyrexia on this admission too, but no physical abnormality had been found after intensive investigations. The illness had cleared up quite quickly with chlorpromazine, leaving few side-effects and, because of a history of cannabis use, a diagnosis of 'possible drug-induced psychosis' had been made.

It was decided to admit Mr Daniels to the intensive-care ward for observation.

The first priority in the successful treatment of a patient is to establish the right kind of relationship. The doctor's courtesy, fellow-feeling, and confidence in the value of psychiatric treatment can help allay apprehension even in a patient as apparently unco-operative as Mr Daniels. Only after this has been done is the next step possible, which is to obtain all the information necessary for accurate diagnosis and successful treatment. Getting this information may take time. For example, the staff only discovered a month after Mr Daniel's admission that his comment that half his brain was linked to the moon was part of a more complex belief that a war was being fought out inside his head between God in the right side of his brain, and the Devil in the other.

Usually a good deal of information about the patient is necessary for optimal psychiatric treatment. This is because the disorder may be manifest in many areas of functioning and all need to be checked. Personal factors such as constitution, character, and social relationships influence the expression of a disorder, as well as the choice of treatment and the prognosis.

This reliance on historical information in psychiatry means that careful record-keeping is particularly important. We have found the following eight principles useful.

1. Clearly indicate whether reports are of observations, e.g. the fact that Mr Daniels had sworn, or judgements, e.g. that this was 'a sure sign of illness'.

2. Make a definite judgement whether information is accurate and if a report is dubious, indicate this clearly. Accuracy may be checked by comparison with another account or with an estimate made by using such characteristics as consistency, credibility, and objectivity. Information known to be false may still sometimes be of value as, for example, when it demonstrates delusional memory or the character of a social relationship.

3. Separate information about history and mental state. History documents how the present state has been reached, but the mental state examination provides selected information about the present state. Observations made by the psychiatrist about the patient should therefore be put into a separate category, often entitled 'Mental state'. This category will also contain reports about the patient's experiences but only (1) if the reports are of the patient's condition in the present or immediate past (2) if they are thought to be accurate and (3) if they concern certain psychological functions which are of particular psychiatric significance. All psychiatrists need to be practised in the assessment of these functions and the questions which probe them. Most psychiatrists follow a standard check-list such as that given in *Notes on eliciting and recording clinical information*, Institute of Psychiatry, Oxford University Press (1973).

4. Provide a separate account of the physical state.

5. Put historical information into categories each incorporating similar information, e.g. 'Complaints' or 'History of the

present illness', and place the categories into a standard order. We follow the order given in *Notes on eliciting and recording clinical information.*

6. Order information within categories chronologically.
7. Summarize information whenever this can be done without making unwarranted assumptions.
8. Record history obtained from other informants separately, quoting the informant's name, relationship to the patient and means of contacting them. The information from several sources can be combined later, in the formulation.

The last five principles are all *organizational* ones, i.e. they relate to how the information is collected and recorded. It is desirable to organize available information from the very first moments of the contact with the patient. Organization brings together related information so that inconsistencies can be ironed out, and irrelevant information discarded. It also makes it possible to locate quickly some sought-for detail.

The emphasis of the history will differ in different patients and in different disorders. A careful history of previous occupation and social relationships will be necessary in someone who is suspected of having a personality disorder but may be much less important in an elderly person with dementia. On the other hand detailed information about the physical layout of the patient's accommodation may be essential in the latter case but not in the former. The importance of the personal context of psychiatric disorder has already been mentioned and will be a consistent theme throughout the book. Individual psychiatrists will also place a slightly different emphasis on what information to collect, e.g. some will stress early life experiences, others family interaction, whilst others again will want information about more remote family members who may have had psychiatric disorders. However, experience has shown that there are broad areas of relevance to diagnosis or treatment in almost all psychiatric patients and these are investigated by experienced psychiatrists of every persuasion. Adopting a particular organizational scheme by learning the sequence of subheadings (such as 'Complaints' or 'Sexual History') and using them consistently is a useful way to ensure that investigation is systematically carried out in each of these areas.

Practical aspects of history-taking

Most interviews begin with the informant giving an account of the problem in the sequence that seems most natural to them. Once they have unburdened themselves it is usually necessary to ask direct questions and these can follow the same order of topics which will be used in writing down the information. This procedure enables the interviewer to be more attentive to the patient rather than worrying about which questions to ask next. Also, since the order of questions is constructed to make sense of the patient's present situation this often gives reassurance that the psychiatrist is trying to get a complete understanding of the patient's problems.

It is often necessary to get information from other sources or on other occasions. Some of the main sources are:

1. Previous notes, notes from other hospitals, and reports, e.g. school reports.
2. Other informants, often a close relative, but sometimes a flat-mate, a neighbour, an employer, or anyone else who can give valuable information about the patient.
3. Observation and closer acquaintance of the patient over a period of time.
4. Additional factual information obtained from the patient.

Omitted from the list are any special investigations or tests that may be carried out.

It is most important to collate this information so that important details do not get overlooked. Here again a standard organizational schema is useful as collation may uncover discrepancies. Usually these arise because of some misunderstanding on the part of the psychiatrist, but sometimes they can be due to deliberate or inadvertent misinformation. One of the commonest reasons for the psychiatrist to be inadvertently misled is when the patient's mood so colours his or her perception of events that the psychiatrist's own judgement is influenced. It is almost always useful, therefore, to collect information from another source to supplement the patient's report. This will be especially important where the report is crucial to the diagnosis or the management.

Initially it is useful to keep information collected from different sources separate but as more information is obtained it is necessary to combine all the information in order to keep hold of the essential elements. Having a familiar sequence of subheadings assists in this process of summarization.

Re-expressing this information in standard terms takes the co-ordination a stage further. It is desirable to do this for brevity and because some agreement can be achieved about what these terms mean within psychiatry. There is wide variation in the everyday usage of all words, but this is particularly true with words describing emotion, even when these appear unambiguous.

It is undesirable to re-label patients' or informants' reports if it is not completely clear what is being reported. One purpose of organizing these reports is, in fact, to show up just such areas of doubt which can then be cleared up in subsequent interviews. The whole of a full psychiatric history cannot be attended to at the same time. If the history is organized, however, the facts of the history will be ordered into categories which build on one another, with facts within each category generally being organized chronologically. The history is then like a narrative. The reader, or listener, can attend to the 'line' or perhaps 'paragraph' that is current and, even though earlier paragraphs become hazy, they have provided enough preparation and background for the current 'paragraph' to be understood and assimilated.

The need for the auditor to have information 'pre-digested' in this fashion if it is to be assimilated is sometimes not understood by examination candidates who give unnecessary irritation to their examiners by not assisting the examiners to grasp the case history.

However, the narrative quality of a well-organized history is not merely an examination device. It provides a sense of the patient's development, the impact of vicissitudes and, occasionally, some incoherence in the narrative points to a hitherto undisclosed event or influence.

It is also the logic of the narrative which determines the order of the subheadings of the history. Any particular moment of a patient's history develops out of earlier events and experiences with which the psychiatrist first needs to become acquainted. The family history therefore precedes the personal history because knowing about previous generations is helpful in understanding the present one. The patient's complaints and sometimes the history of the present illness come first because, like the introduction to a book, these state the purpose of the enquiry. The description of personality comes last in the history, just before the mental state, because this is, in a sense, a summary of certain regularities in the previous history, and is another lens through which the current mental state is viewed.

The process of organizing a history is particularly well illustrated in the case of Mr Daniels who could not give one during the first week of his admission; information was obtained in a piecemeal and unco-ordinated fashion. We anticipate that our readers will either find this history difficult to grasp as presented, or will begin to organize it in their minds in order to obtain the essential facts. We recommend that readers write out the same history in an organized fashion, using the headings given in *Notes on eliciting and recording clinical information* before reading our history which follows below.

Below is a summary of the information obtained on Mr Daniels.

Summary

Presenting complaint

From patient: None available, mute. Mr Ernest Daniels was referred by day centre staff who were concerned about his disturbed behaviour.
From mother: A two-week history of increasing disturbed behaviour characterized by restlessness, violent outbursts, and odd ideas.
From day centre: Several days of increasingly odd and socially inappropriate behaviour associated with the expressed belief that he was dead and that half his brain was linked to the moon.

Past psychiatric history

One previous admission for possibly drug-induced psychosis associated with pyrexia.

Mental state examination

Mute young man who appeared hostile and suspicious of the examiner and kept his eyes shut during the interview. He occasionally shouted 'no' but otherwise had no spontaneous speech. He did understand and respond to spoken requests.

Physical examination

Pyrexial (T= 38.5) with tachycardia (120 beats per minute).

Further information

Mr Daniels had first been in hospital the previous year but had had no previous serious physical illnesses. During his stay in hospital he complained that people smelt like rotten pork and also believed that he had special powers. He had similar thoughts on his present admission: occasionally thinking that people smelt like dead pigs and also that he was one of the few chosen to have a special mark on his forehead (actually a self-inflicted abrasion). On this admission he also believed that his breathing had altered and that his body had changed from 'soft' to 'strong'. He thought that people around him were 'the Devil' and that the Devil was trying to gain control of one half of his brain which was linked to the moon.

Mr Daniels' mother was a 42-year-old laundry worker who had had several admissions to a psychiatric hospital with a diagnosis of schizophrenia. She continued to have fluphenazine depot injections. She reported that Mr Daniels had had a normal full-term birth in Guyana, but had had pneumonia in infancy. Mrs Daniels had gone back to work when he was 12 months old and when he was three had come to England to join her husband who was a 52-year-old caretaker. The couple had five other children: Alan aged nine, Joyce, 23, an unmarried mother, Winston, 18, Stella, 15, and Pat, 16. The three youngest children were still at home.

Mr Daniels had been brought up by his maternal grandmother until he was nine years old, when he came to join his parents in the UK. He had not attended school in Guyana and could not write when he went to English secondary school. He did well in a remedial class but could not get work after leaving school. Eventually he did a carpentry course and got a job as a carpenter, but was sacked after 10 days. His only subsequent work had been in a hospital rehabilitation unit.

Before his previous admission he had become very interested in Rastafarianism and then Islam. He had smoked cannabis heavily but denied smoking cannabis before the present admission. When he was examined he was sweaty, feverish and had a tachycardia. He was initially mute but when he began to speak it was apparent that he was fully orientated and there was no evidence of any cognitive abnormality. Routine drug screening was negative. He denied hearing voices. His sleep was disturbed but there was no other evidence of mood disturbance. He did say that people could look through his forehead into his brain but denied that they could read or interfere with his thoughts. However on another occasion he did say that the Devil could switch on his left-hand 'evil' brain at will. When first admitted he would refuse to answer questions or would shout 'no'. His behaviour was unpredictable, e.g. he would suddenly run down the ward and kick the entrance door. Mr Daniels gave few details about the time leading up to this admission but his mother did give the history already described. She and Mr Daniels seemed to get on well although she worried that he had never had a girlfriend and thought that her husband was too hard on him. She was also worried about his violent and unpredictable behaviour.

Further summary of Mr Daniels, aged 17

Presenting complaint (from mother and day centre staff)

Appeared well until two weeks before admission when he had seemed restless.

One week before there were definite signs of relapse and he had threatened his father. He had wanted at this time to come back to the hospital. He had started to say that half his brain was linked to the moon at the day centre.

Two days before admission he had smashed furniture at his parents' home, and just before admission had disrupted a staff meeting at the day centre.

Family history

Mother: aged 52, laundry worker. Under treatment for schizophrenia. Came to England with father when Mr Daniels was three years old.

Father: aged 52, caretaker. Conflict in relationship with patient.

Siblings: Joyce, 23, unmarried mother with a baby daughter, shares flat with patient; Winston, 18, unmarried; the patient, 17; Pat, 16, lives at home; Stella, 15, lives at home; Alan, nine, lives at home. Mother only family member with psychiatric disorder.

Personal history

Born in Guyana. Full-term, normal delivery. Brought up by maternal grandmother from 12 months old until aged nine when he came to live with parents in an inner city area in a large northern city.

Education: Age 11–16: comprehensive school. Remedial class.
     Age 16: three months course in carpentry.

Occupation: Age 17: ten days as a carpenter. Sacked because of rudeness.

Sexual history: No heterosexual relationship. Nil else known.

Drug use: Heavy use of cannabis when aged 16 but nil recently.

Past medical history

Pneumonia when nine months old.
Pyrexia of unknown origin when aged 16.

Past psychiatric history

Psychotic illness when aged 16: three month history of religious preoccupations and heavy cannabis use. Olfactory hallucinations and grandiose ideas noted.

Previous personality

No information.

Mental state examination

Appearance and general behaviour

Initially mute, then would shout 'no' when asked to do things.

Behaviour explosive on first admission with sudden outbursts of violent activity.

Talk

Mute at first. Later, he began to talk spontaneously and then answered questions promptly and sensibly.

Mood

Not depressed or elated. No appetite disturbance. Reduction of total sleep time.

Thought content

Preoccupied by his abnormal ideas.

Abnormal beliefs and interpretation of events

Believes that he is one of the chosen few, that abrasion on his forehead demonstrates this and that his bodily functions have altered. Thinking that his brain can be 'looked into' but denies that thoughts can be read. Believes that one side of his brain could be controlled by the Devil.

Abnormal experiences

Occasional olfactory hallucinations (smell of dead pigs coming from people). Denies auditory hallucinations.

Cognitive state

Normal.

Attention, concentration and memory

No abnormality detected.

Intelligence

Low or low to average.

Appraisal of illness

Convinced of the reality of his experiences.

Physical examination

Abrasion on forehead. Sweating. Reluctant to be examined. $T = 38.5°C$, $P = 120$ per minute, full and regular.

We have now reached the stage of history and examination with which subsequent chapters of this book will begin. In doing so, we have not discussed many aspects of obtaining information, such as interview technique, but we have shown how many disparate pieces of information can be organized.

Organization is not an end in itself but has practical value. Making a diagnosis is one such but it is not the only one. Learning the circumstances and previous experiences of a patient also adds to the understanding of the impact of the illness and to the prediction of the response to a particular treatment. Consequently, psychiatrists often think about or describe patients' problems in the form of a short synopsis which contains personal information about the patient as well as likely diagnoses, possible causes, suggested lines of treatment and thoughts about prognosis.

These synopses, or formulations, are a further step in the organization of the information about the patient. They contain what the psychiatrist keeps in mind from the full summary because it seems most important to his management of the case. The ability to make the right selection, or inference, is one of the essential skills of psychiatry. There are no rules to say what is right for a particular case but we have tried to illustrate the process in this book. What is right will depend, in any case, on why the information is wanted. However, we have generally found that formulations have to be continually made and then modified in the attempt to answer three closely related questions.

1. 'Are there any ambiguities or gaps in my knowledge?' 'Do I need to get more information'?
2. 'Is there information about which I am doubtful?' 'Do I need to get it clarified?'
3. 'What are the psychiatric implications of this information?' 'What is the diagnosis, or treatment, or prognosis?'

We have found it helpful to make and test tentative formulations from very early on in an interview with a patient. This not only makes taking a history a much more active and enquiring process, it is also a comfort if something unexpected or urgent happens, because the interviewer has ready a view of the underlying problem. We have tried to show in subsequent chapters how an initial formulation gradually becomes modified as gaps in information are filled, doubts clarified and the results of action taken become apparent.

We end this chapter with a summary, followed by the first provisional formulation of Mr Daniels' illness. This formulation, sketchy as it was, was particularly important when Mr Daniels absconded shortly after admission, because it enabled the staff to recognize that Mr Daniels was both psychotic and a danger to others and so led to effective action.

Short summary

Mr Daniels is a 17-year-old Guyanese man. He was seen as an emergency after a short history of unusually aggressive and inexplicable behaviour, and abnormal ideas.

Mr Daniels had been mainly brought up by his maternal grand-mother but does not appear to have experienced emotional problems on leaving her and coming to this country to join his parents and five siblings at the age of nine. He needed remedial teaching at school and failed to obtain regular work. There is therefore a possibility that he is mildly subnormal in intelligence. He has had a previous episode of a similar illness which was preceded by heavy cannabis use but there is no evidence of this on this occasion and drug screen is negative.

Noteworthy features of his present mental state are olfactory hallucinations and complex grandiose and religious delusions which include the belief that his brain can be controlled by the Devil. There are no definite features of mood disturbance and no cognitive impairment. However an atypical feature is a pyrexia which was also found on his previous admission.

Formulation

Diagnosis

Mr Daniels is psychotic.

Although mute on admission, he was not stuporose and was found not to be confused when this could be conclusively tested. An acute brain syndrome, which may have been suggested by his pyrexia, can therefore be ruled out.

There are no features of an affective disorder, but there are many features of schizophrenia, including a delusion of passivity. Schizophrenia, or a schizophreniform illness, is therefore the most likely diagnosis.

Aetiology

Mr Daniels has both a family history of schizophrenia and a previous history of an illness similar to the present one. It should therefore be assumed that he has a long-standing vulnerability to schizophrenia.

The previous illness was associated with heavy cannabis use, and may have been drug-induced. The history is against drug-induction of this illness, but this cannot yet be excluded.

The marked pyrexia suggests an occult physical disorder of which psychosis may be symptomatic, but despite extensive investigations no disorder was found on the previous admission, when Mr Daniels was also pyrexial. It is possible that the pyrexia on this occasion is a manifestation of an unusually severe degree of the physiological response that may occur in the first few days of an acute psychosis.

The conflict in Mr Daniels' family during the early part of his illness suggests that family factors may be important in explaining the severity of his breakdown.

Further investigations

More information on Mr Daniels' recent drug intake needs to be obtained. His physical state needs to be thoroughly investigated. Other precipitants of this present illness, such as stresses in his home situation or recent life-events, should not be neglected whilst these investigations are progressing since several synergistic factors may have been active. In the longer term the satisfactoriness of Mr Daniels' social involvement between his two illnesses will need to be assessed. If his family is an important source of support to him, even though he left home, their attitude to his illness and to him will need to be investigated.

Management

Mr Daniels has been violent before admission and in-patient treatment is indicated. Neuroleptic treatment has been effective in the past and is likely to be so again. Little would be gained by further observation of him without medication, and to do so would increase the risk of violence on the ward and would also add unnecessary difficulty to the task of making a relationship and obtaining a history from Mr Daniels.

If he initially refuses treatment every attempt should be made to persuade him otherwise before a compulsory treatment order, which would be applicable in this case, is invoked.

Further treatment should be based on the determination of the cause of the present illness.

Prognosis

The prognosis for this episode is likely to be good, as it was for the previous epidsode. Longer-term prognosis will depend on the final diagnosis.

2

The importance of a detailed and careful enquiry in evaluating suicidal risk—the case of Arthur Wrigley, aged 59

The history, as it was first recorded in out-patients, was as follows.

Presenting complaint

Mr Wrigley was referred by his general practitioner for an urgent out-patient assessment. The letter said, in part, 'he is suffering anxiety depression and has suicidal tendencies. He wanted to assault himself with a knife last April [five months before] . . . his depression is getting worse and I am quite concerned about him'. Mr Wrigley was seen on his own, and his account was as follows. He complained that he was a 'whole mass of nerves' and that he 'just couldn't keep still'.

He was 'stopping away from people' which was 'not like me'. Mr Wrigley dated these symptoms from his retirement on medical grounds. Two years before the interview he had 'a stroke' affecting his right side. He made a good recovery but two months later he had another on his left side leaving him with a weak arm and leg. Although it 'soon wore off' this resulted in his having to give up his job as a hospital porter since he was no longer thought to be capable of heavy lifting. No alternative employment was available and he was made redundant.

Mr Wrigley felt himself to be increasingly 'changed' after that. He began to burst into tears over nothing, felt that he had to force himself to eat because he had no appetite for food and slept for shorter and shorter periods at night. He lost interest in sex, and he and his wife had not had sexual intercourse for 18 months before the interview. His wife had taken to sleeping in a separate bed because of his restlessness at night.

As mentioned in the general practitioner's letter, Mr Wrigley reported that he had made an attempt on his life five months before. He said that he had been having tea with his daughter, his wife, and her sister and picked up a knife from the table and made as if to stab himself with it. He had burst into anguished tears when he was restrained, and sobbed, 'I'm sorry, I'm sorry'.

His general practitioner had treated him with benzodiazepines but Mr Wrigley felt little benefit from them. He had been told that he could not drink alcohol whilst taking them. Since he felt that it was not manly to drink soft drinks, he had avoided social occasions and so became more socially isolated.

Family history

Mr Wrigley's father died when Mr Wrigley was one year old. He could remember nothing about him. His mother died some years before his illness. He described her as a capable, cheerful lady.

Mr Wrigley was the youngest of three siblings. His brother died of a brain tumour at the age of 20 when Mr Wrigley was 19. A sister had died a few months before the interview.

Mr Wrigley gave no family history of psychiatric disorder or epilepsy.

Personal history

Mr Wrigley's had been, he said, a happy childhood. He was born and brought up in a close-knit, but impoverished area of inner London. He enjoyed school, leaving at 14 without qualifications. Mr Wrigley found work immediately after leaving school and was continuously employed, excluding a period of war service, in various jobs until his early retirement. His occupations had all involved labouring or assembly work.

Mr Wrigley married at the age of 28 and had two children, a son and a daughter. He described his marriage as happy. He lived in a council flat with his wife and daughter.

Past medical history

Mr Wrigley had two recent cerebro-vascular episodes as already described, but could not recall any other serious illness.

Past psychiatric history

Mr Wrigley had a period of in-patient treatment whilst in the forces during the Second World War. It was assumed that this was associated with depression following the death of his brother.

Previous personality

Mr Wrigley's account of himself suggested that before his illness he was optimistic, active, and sociable with no tendency to get depressed.

Mental state examination

Appearance and general behaviour

Mr Wrigley was a tall, greying, notably thin man who showed no spontaneous movements and whose face was set in an expression of both sadness and apprehension. He seemed often on the point of tears.

Talk

Mr Wrigley spoke slowly and with no tonal modulation. He was markedly slow in replying to questions. His answers were to the point but terse.

Mood

Mr Wrigley felt and appeared agitated and miserable. There was nothing he enjoyed and he had to force himself to eat. He had lost over 14 lb (6 kg) in weight since the beginning of his illness. He lay awake for up to two hours after going to bed at night and usually woke again after two or three hours and was then unable to get back to sleep. He had lost interest in all his customary activities (betting, sing-song evenings at the club and gardening at home) but his energy was little affected and he spent a great deal of his day on long solitary walks. He reported difficulty in concentrating and could not sit and watch television. He also had difficulty in remembering things, for example, the names of friends and the words of songs. He had lost all interest in sex.

Mr Wrigley said that he felt that life was not worth living. He had wished to die and occasionally thought of ending his life, but had made no plans to do so and said that he had no current intention of ending his life.

Thought content

Mr Wrigley had vague worries about his health. His main pre-occupation was with his lost work. He felt that he would never have become ill if he had only stayed at work.

Abnormal beliefs and interpretation of events

None were elicited.

Cognitive state

Mr Wrigley was orientated in space and knew the day, month, and year, although not the date. His recall of a name and address after five minutes was perfect. Mr Wrigley was asked about current news items and accurately reported two.

Appraisal of illness

Mr Wrigley said that 'my nerves have been affected by my inability to adapt to retirement'.

Physical examination

Not performed.

Mr Wrigley's wife and youngest daughter were briefly interviewed and confirmed the broad outlines of the history of the presenting complaint and of the previous psychiatric history. Their description of Mr Wrigley's personality was consistent with the one that he had given. Mrs Wrigley wanted her husband 'to have some treatment'. She was angry with her general practitioner for his reluctance to refer her husband to a psychiatrist earlier. This referral had only come about, she said, because she had 'threatened to go private'.

Neither Mr nor Mrs Wrigley wanted him to come into hospital.

Summary

Mr Wrigley is a 59-year-old retired hospital porter who was seen in the out-patient department at the request of his general practitioner. He is a married man with two children, the younger of whom still lives with his wife and himself. He was born and had been brought up in the local area. His father died when he was aged one. One brother died when he was 20 and a sister had died recently. The patient was briefly 'depressed' after his brother died but had no other psychiatric illness and appears to have been a consistently cheerful and sociable man.

Two years ago he had a stroke affecting his right side, and subsequently another stroke affecting his left side which resulted in his being retired from work on medical grounds. Since then he has become increasingly preoccupied with his loss and has come to regard the future with hopelessness. Over the last 18 months, he has lost over 14 lbs (6 kg) in weight and has woken early in the morning. His personality has also changed considerably, in that he has gradually given up his interests and has avoided meeting other people. He has made a suicide attempt five months previously.

When seen, he was anxious and dejected. He was retarded in speech but his concentration and memory were not clinically impaired and he was not deluded or hallucinated. He has thought of ending his life but has no plans to do so.

It is fairly clear that Mr Wrigley is depressed. Uppermost in the psychiatrist's mind, in assessing a depressed, unemployed man in late middle-age, will be the risk of suicide. The psychiatrist has to decide how serious this risk is before terminating the interview.

Formulation

Diagnosis

Mr Wrigley has a physical handicap resulting from his two recent cerebrovascular episodes but he also has an independent psychological disorder whose main feature is depression. Some degree of depression is understandable, although by no means inevitable, after severe illness. This should not prevent the diagnosis of a depressive disorder. The first point to be considered therefore, is whether Mr Wrigley is experiencing a prolonged depressive reaction to either his stroke, or his redundancy. However, adjustment reactions rarely last as long as 18 months, and do not increase in severity as Mr Wrigley's condition has done. Mr Wrigley seems in fact to be suffering from an illness in which the range of normal adjustments is exceeded, for example, by his symptoms of persistent biological change, such as sleep disturbance and weight loss. His state has also become autonomous, as illnesses do, and has not been ameliorated by the recovery from his strokes with the passage of time. This is all evidence in favour of Mr Wrigley having a depressive illness. The severity of his condition justifies a diagnosis of depressive psychosis, rather than one of depressive neurosis.

Aetiology

Three types of aetiological factors must be considered:

1. Predisposing (or vulnerability) factors
2. Provoking factors
3. Exacerbating factors

It is convenient to split each of these into (a) biological, and (b) psychosocial components.

Since relatively little personal information is available about Mr Wrigley none of the possible aetiological factors can be ruled out at this stage and each of them will therefore be considered.

1(a) *Biological predisposition (constitution)*

Although most individuals have the capacity to become depressed it is supposed by many psychiatrists that a few have a hereditary disposition to do so more severely, or in response to less extreme and more wide-ranging challenges. As already noted, Mr Wrigley gives little evidence of this depressive 'diathesis': there is no known family history of depression or 'depressive spectrum' disorder such as alcoholism, which occurs more commonly in relatives of patients with a hereditary predisposition to depression. Neither does Mr Wrigley have a depressive, anankastic or cyclothymic personality which are also associated with a possible hereditary, predisposition to depression.

1(b) Psychosocial predisposition (early experience)

The details of Mr Wrigley's early upbringing so far available are insufficiently detailed to assess its contribution but it has been suggested that individuals who have lost a parent by death in infancy, as has Mr Wrigley, are more likely to develop depression in later life.

2(a) Biological provocation (recent illness)

Strokes are known to provoke depression. Having a stroke is frightening in the short-term and may cause grief in the longer-term because of the loss of physical function that it causes. However, depression may also be a direct consequence of neurological impairment, particularly when this involves limbic structures.

2(b) Psychosocial provocation (adverse life-events)

Although a wide variety of life-experiences may provoke depression, those involving threat or loss appear to be the most noxious. Mr Wrigley has experienced three major events involving loss—his redundancy, his stroke and the later loss of his sister—and one of these also carries with it a threat of future serious disability or death (the stroke). Each of these events are likely to have many subsidiary consequences, and these, too, may provoke further depression. One example given by Mr Wrigley is that he engaged less in one of his principle sources of pleasure, going to the 'club' with his friends, because he was ashamed of being redundant and because he had difficulty in remembering the words of the songs that were sung in the bar.

3(a) Biological exacerbation (physical disability)

This may have an indirect effect. Any persistent disability after the stroke may restrict or prevent activities which would normally be recuperative. Very little is known about Mr Wrigley's physical state but it is known that his stroke lost him his job and that unemployment generally results in a reduced ability to cope with adversity.

3(b) *Psychosocial exacerbation (coping strategies and resources)*

It is not known which strategies Mr Wrigley used to surmount difficulty, nor what help was available to him through relationships with other people, notably his wife. However, if much of Mr Wrigley's self-esteem and the esteem of others comes from his skills at doing a job and earning a wage then he is likely to cope worse with both redundancy and physical disability than someone who experiences themselves as valued for some other attribute, such as sensitivity to others.

Further investigations

Mr Wrigley is suffering from a depressive psychosis, and although his is not presently deluded or hallucinated, examination of his mental state at a later date might reveal these abnormalities.

More information is needed to determine the aetiology of Mr Wrigley's illness. In a first out-patient interview it is difficult to obtain a full family and personal history but it will be necessary to obtain this at a later stage in order to test some of the aetiological hypotheses already mentioned. The diagnosis of manic-depressive psychosis could be more confidently ruled out if this failed to reveal evidence of a manic-depressive diathesis. It will be necessary, for example, to inquire further about the emotional atmosphere in Mr Wrigley's family of origin, their material circumstances, and his memories of or thoughts about his father, and about his reaction to his mother's death. It would be helpful to know more about his marriage and his relationship with his children.

More enquiry needs to be made about his neurological disability since the stroke. More detailed cognitive testing and a physical examination should be performed. A CT scan may be indicated to determine the sites of the cerebral lesions, and assess their size.

Mr Wrigley's ability to cope needs to be assessed. It is convenient to do this by considering his personal resources and his social and material resources separately. His personal history is likely to be a particularly good gauge of the former. How he responded to previous losses and how he tried to combat the depression in its early stages are two considerations. Mr Wrigley's major social resources are his wife and his friends at the club. Some assessment needs to be made of the present quality of these relationships, and how much support Mr Wrigley feels he receives from these. Something needs to be known about his home, whether he owns it, how satisfactory it is to him and his contact with his neighbours. It is often useful to enquire specifically about debts.

The timing of the events leading up to Mr Wrigley's illness also needs to be checked against the development of his symptoms since this will give crucial information about which of the possible factors precipitated his depressive illness.

The information so far considered has not been essential to immediate management, and can therefore be obtained at a later date. However some information necessary for confidently determining immediate management is missing and this is considered in the next session.

Management

The most pressing problem is whether or not Mr Wrigley should come into hospital, in order to expedite his treatment, to relieve his distress and, most urgently, to prevent suicide or serious self-harm resulting from a failed suicide attempt. The answer depends on the characteristics of Mr Wrigley's illness, his intentions, his previous behaviour, and his personal situation.

The first step in the management is therefore to review these characteristics, especially those that are risk factors for suicide, and to enquire further about those whose presence is still undetermined.

Intentions and previous behaviour

Mr Wrigley was clear that he had considered suicide but had made no plans to carry this out. Considerable importance is usually attached to the patient's intentions, and supplementary questions (such as 'have you ever thought how you would kill yourself') should also be put. There are indications that Mr Wrigley minimized his symptoms. It is also possible that he felt that he 'shouldn't have' suicidal ideas and was therefore minimizing these. Even if Mr Wrigley stated his intentions correctly, the weight to put on them will depend on his personality. Impulsive patients may not deliberate for some time about suicide.

The fact that Mr Wrigley has made a previous suicide attempt during the course of the illness is, by contrast, a definite risk factor which should therefore be set against his stated intention not to do so again. Not enough of the circumstances of this attempt is known to be able to assess its seriousness. The exact details need to be enquired into, and it may also be useful to ask the relatives about any other attempts, or apparent preparations for suicide.

Personal situation

Mr Wrigley's age and sex are risk factors: suicide is commonest in men over 50. His lack of employment is also a risk factor, especially because work has, in the past, been a source of both pride and satisfaction to Mr Wrigley.

Mr Wrigley's close ties with family and friends are protective factors. However he has apparently withdrawn socially following the development of his depression and it would be important to establish how much contact he presently has with others, how satisfying this is to him, and to determine how protective these relationships are. It is particularly important to assess the present quality of his relationship with his wife. This should be done tactfully but in some depth, for example by asking about when they last had a row, what it was about, and when they last had any physical contact.

The fact that Mr Wrigley is unwell, that there is an effective treatment, that he is likely to get better more quickly in hospital than at home, and that there are risks to his safety if he remains at home, are all indications for admission to hospital. The risk of suicide is also likely to be reduced by hospital admission, first, because Mr Wrigley could be supervised more closely by nursing staff, secondly, because he might find it easier to disclose suicidal ideas to emotionally neutral, professional care-givers who, anyway, have more experience of the indications which are sometimes given of a suicide attempt, and thirdly, more active treatment can be instituted. Hospital admission would also have the advantage that Mr Wrigley could be removed from any psychosocial factors perpetuating his depression, such as the criticism from families which commonly occurs in response to long-standing irritability or social withdrawal.

It is possible that Mr and Mrs Wrigley will both be worried by this possibility of admission. Mrs Wrigley may feel that she has failed her husband, and Mr Wrigley that he is inadequate or incurable. These, and other worries, must be discussed. Mr and Mrs Wrigley are likely also to want to know about the alternatives to hospital, such as day hospital or out-patient attendance.

Mr Wrigley has suffered from a long illness, his previous suicide attempt occurred five months before his attendance at the hospital, and he attended for a non-urgent out-patient assessment. Should neither he nor his wife be willing for him to come into hospital, the immediate risk to himself is not great enough to justify compulsory admission. However he is ill enough, and the longer-term risk is great enough, for regular, frequent reassessment to be indicated. This could take place most effectively in a day hospital, but could, if necessary, also be done on an out-patient basis, by giving Mr Wrigley an appointment for every two or three days.

Regular reassessment would impress Mr Wrigley with the psychiatrist's concern, it would enable him to build up a lasting relationship with the psychiatrist and to acclimatize himself to the hospital, and it would also help the psychiatrist to gain a more complete understanding of Mr Wrigley and his illness.

The psychiatrist should advise Mr and Mrs Wrigley to contact him immediately should there be any deterioration in Mr Wrigley's condition and should give them an alternative person to contact, should he not be available.

Compulsory admission should be considered if Mr Wrigley continues to refuse hospital admission and his symptoms worsen or if he expresses suicidal ideas. Compulsory admission should also be considered if Mr Wrigley fails to attend for follow-up, but no action should be taken until a home visit has been made.

Once the circumstances in which Mr Wrigley is to be treated have been established the specific elements of the treatment can be considered. The next of these is physical treatment.

Electroconvulsive therapy (ECT) is at least as effective in psychotic depression as drug treatment, and usually quicker. It is contra-indicated, however, if Mr Wrigley's strokes were due to hypertension or bleeding from a vascular malformation and should not therefore be given until Mr Wrigley has been more thoroughly investigated physically. It is also unwise to give the first ever ECT on an out-patient basis. Antidepressant treatment is also likely to be effective since Mr Wrigley appears not to be deluded and at this stage is the treatment of first choice. The dose can be built up more rapidly and side-effects monitored more easily if Mr Wrigley is in hospital, or if he is attending the hospital frequently.

A sedative antidepressant of proven efficacy but safe in over-dose would be best, with the dose being given at night to help Mr Wrigley sleep. Mr Wrigley could also be offered a benzodiaze-pine at night for additional sedation. A relatively long-acting one should be chosen which would continue to give sedation in the early hours of the morning. Mr and Mrs Wrigley should be told that antidepressants may cause a transient worsening of mood shortly after they are begun, and that they take at least two weeks to be fully effective. Patients who respond to antidepressants may become more energetic before they become less depressed. The risk of suicide may consequently be greater during this period, and even more careful supervision necessary.

The risk of suicide must be discussed with Mrs Wrigley and possible warning signs, such as the expression of suicidal ideas, a worsening of his mood or, paradoxically, a sudden elation, should be mentioned.

Discussion of Mrs Wrigley's feelings about the situation may be therapeutic for Mr Wrigley because it may reduce tension between them.

Follow-up visits by Mr Wrigley could also be used to identify and challenge some of his gloomy depressive ruminations—for example, that he has been on the 'scrap heap' since he lost his job.

Prognosis

Assuming that suicide or serious self-harm can be avoided, the prognosis for an episode, such as this one, of depression associ-ated with early morning waking and other biological features is good. This is especially so in view of Mr Wrigley's previous good psychological health. However the chance of relapse, and the longer term prognosis, will depend on how effectively the provoking and exacerbating factors of the current episode can be remedied.

Brief formulation

Mr Wrigley is a 59-year-old married, ex-hospital porter made redundant after a stroke two years ago. He had a second stroke soon after and became increasingly more miserable subsequently. He made a suicide attempt 5 months before this assessment, has lost about 14 lbs (6 kg) in weight and has persistent early morning waking. He appeared depressed at examination and was retarded in speech, but is not deluded or hallucinated.

Diagnosis

Mr Wrigley has a depressive illness. His symptoms border on those of both depressive neurosis and depressive psychosis but in view of the severity of his illness the latter is the more appropriate diagnosis. Of the two diagnoses of depressive psychosis that could apply to Mr Wrigley manic-depressive psychosis, depressed type, is less likely than reactive depressive psychosis.

Aetiology

Constitutional and early environment factors have not been adequately researched although it has been noted that his father died when he was one. Information is also needed about his physical disability, and his ability to cope with adversity. Both his strokes and his retirement are likely to have played some part in provoking his depression.

Further investigations

Background information about Mr Wrigley is lacking. More information is especially needed about possible risk-factors of suicide—the severity of his illness, the quality of his mood, his intentions, the circumstances of his previous suicide attempt, and his personal situation.

Management

There is a significant risk of suicide and hospital admission is advisable. Treatment with a sedative antidepressant and, if he would find it helpful, a benzodiazepine hypnotic should be begun immediately. Frequent reassessment should take place during the early stages of treatment. There are no present grounds for compulsory admission, but this should be considered if Mr Wrigley refuses admission and if his condition deteriorates or he fails to attend for follow-up.

Advice and support of Mrs Wrigley should not be neglected. She should be advised of the risk of suicide and if Mr Wrigley is not admitted to hospital, she should be recommended to contact the doctor immediately if Mr Wrigley should seem to be deteriorating, or if he should begin to express suicidal ideas. Cognitive therapy may be a helpful adjunct to Mr Wrigley's management.

Prognosis

The prognosis for this episode is good providing that Mr Wrigley does not harm himself. Future prognosis will depend to a large extent on the resolution of his concern about his stroke and his redundancy.

Further information

Mr Wrigley could not be persuaded to come into hospital and made light of his depression. He was given an out-patient appointment, but for two weeks later. A tricyclic antidepressant dothiepin, was also started, initially at a dose of 75 mg at night and then increasing after a week to 125 mg at night.

On the day that he was next due to be seen Mr Wrigley cut his throat and both his wrists with a blade from a safety razor. He left the following note on two blank pages torn out of a book.

To Doris (wife) and Tracey (daughter)

I just can't take any more of this misery I feel and I am making your life and Trasey's a misery to. That is the way I feel from morning till night. I've had enough so I'm getting out of it. I am sorry love. That is the way I feel. I leave the money in the bank to you Dorris. And the money upstairs under my shirts. I can't take any more Dorris. Nor can you. If we can't live happy it's NO GOOD. I'm making life A MISERY for you and Trasey. I'm sorry, good bye love. I want to be cremated Dorris.

PS Tell Lofty and my other mates that they're THE BEST FRIENDS anyone could have.

He was semi-conscious when discovered by his daughter and was subsequently admitted to hospital, where he was found to have severed his long flexor tendons and his ulnar artery in his left wrist and to have incised his larynx at his neck. Other vital structures had been missed, as often occurs if the throat is cut when the neck is extended. The skin of his right wrist was cut in a number of places but deeper structures were untouched. Mr Wrigley's systolic blood pressure on admission was 60. He was resuscitated and an emergency tracheotomy was performed. The severed tendons were repaired and his wounds sutured. An in-dwelling urinary catheter was also inserted.

Mr Wrigley's physical condition rapidly improved and four days later he was seen by the same psychiatrist who had seen him in the out-patient department. Mr Wrigley's first remarks to him were an apology for what he had done, and a reassurance that 'it wasn't your fault'. He said that he was sorry that he had failed and wanted to be dead, but 'would never do that again. Not after all the work you doctors have done'. Mr Wrigley was transferred to the psychiatric unit shortly after, and the nurse accompanying him reported that he was 'much better' and was smiling. Mr Wrigley's physical convalescence was uneventful, apart from an acute exacerbation of his chronic bronchitis which responded to physiotherapy and antibiotics. His most persistent physical complaint was the weakness of his right hand.

The nursing staff were particularly anxious about Mr Wrigley making another suicide attempt. When asked whether he had any intention to do so he would say 'I think I've done enough damage' and then smile or make a joke. He was seen to bang his right hand on furniture and described his physical condition as 'rubbish'. On one visit by his wife and daughter he alarmed them by picking up a knife and stroking its edge with his thumb for several minutes.

Mr Wrigley's antidepressant was restarted after his transfer from the surgical ward, and chlorpromazine added at night. Mrs Wrigley and her daughter were interviewed again, and a more detailed history obtained from Mr Wrigley after his tracheotomy tube had been removed, and he could talk without undue strain. The recorded history was as follows.

Little new information was obtained about Mr Wrigley's father. Mr Wrigley had no memory of him and had never enquired about him. He thought he died in his late 30s and that he had a bad chest and possible tuberculosis. His mother died aged 91 from 'old age'. His younger sister, who had died earlier that year, had had a 'nervous breakdown' in the 1930s but no further information was available. She had remained unmarried until she was 50 and had no children. He confirmed that his family had always been close. He regularly saw his own children, and kept in touch with his sister's son who was in Australia.

Mr Wrigley's various jobs included furnace labouring, and motor mower assembly. He had been a hospital porter for 10 years, since leaving the Water Board with whom he had been a labourer. He married at 29 after a courtship of only three months. His wife was four years older than himself. Mrs Wrigley described the marriage as 'generally happy' and said that they had the 'occasional row'. She said that Mr Wrigley had always been affectionate with the children but did not enjoy their company particularly. She described herself as 'nervy' and said that she had recently developed asthma.

Mrs Wrigley usually described her husband as 'daft' when talking about his suicide attempt. She spoke much more than he did in interviews, and on one occasion said 'I know about depression. No-one has been more depressed than I have'.

The Wrigley's son was married. Tracey, their daughter, was 20, lived at home and had been unemployed since leaving school. Both children were very concerned about their father and visited regularly.

Mr Wrigley was a heavy smoker. He drank most nights and went to the pub several days a week; this had become his main interest in the last few years. His family concurred in saying that before his illness he had been a very sociable, well-liked, and equable man who preferred the company of other men.

Some further details were added to the history of Mr Wrigley's illness. He retired after his first stroke but his mood remained cheerful until his second stroke, two months later. His general practitioner considered that he was 'understandably upset' about losing his job and had been reluctant to treat him. Mr Wrigley reinforced this view by dismissing his psychological symptoms in consultations, which were usually for physical symptoms such as 'stabbing pain' in his side or 'funny feelings' in his epigastrium.

No history of medical illness previous to Mr Wrigley's strokes was obtained. He had been investigated by a neurologist following the second stroke. The medical notes were obtained and it was found that Mr Wrigley was then noted to have increased tone in all four limbs, greater on the left than the right. His cardiovascular system was normal, and he was not hypertensive. Aortography showed a common origin of the subclavian and carotid arteries but was otherwise normal. The CT scan showed a small radiolucent area adjacent to the lateral border of the body of the right ventricle, which did not enhance after the injection of radiopaque material. There was no other abnormality.

A diagnosis of brain-stem ischaemia had been made and Mr Wrigley was discharged on aspirin. Mr Wrigley did not continue this believing that he could not drink while taking it. His depressed mood was noted at out-patient follow-up, but his complaints of pain and weight loss were thought to be physical in origin.

Ten days after transfer to the psychiatric unit Mr Wrigley's physical condition was as follows. He was fully mobile. He still had a small sinus over the site of his tracheotomy but there was no communication with his trachea. His neck and wrists had healed, and his chest was clear. His cardiovascular system was normal, and he was passing water normally. No abnormalities of his facial nerves were demonstrable. He had full movement and power in his left hand but the tone was increased and power significantly reduced in his right, dominant hand. He could not oppose his right thumb to any of his fingers. Power was normal in both legs. Reflexes were brisk in his right arm with scapular and finger jerks both being present. Other reflexes were normal. He had agraphaesthesia and astereognosis of both hands which was worse on the right than the left. He complained of his right hand being 'dead', but light touch sensation was only mildly impaired, and pin-prick sensation was normal.

When he was interviewed at a ward round 10 days after transfer, Mr Wrigley looked pale and listless, but his face betrayed little emotion except for a fixedly corrugated forehead and occasional moistening of his eyes. He smiled once or twice in response to his own 'jokes'—for example, when his wife's concern for him was being discussed, he said 'she's only interested while she doesn't know where I keep my money'.

Mr Wrigley's spirits appeared to improve shortly after his transfer but then sank again, although he still said that 'he was slightly better than last year'. His appetite was still poor, but his sleep had returned to normal. He said 'not yet' when asked whether he had again thought of ending his life: and he prefaced discussions about the future with his family with the proviso 'if I'm still here'. There was no diurnal variation of his mood.

On several occasions Mr Wrigley expressed abnormally suspicious ideas. For example, in a casual conversation in the hospital grounds he said that everyone in his neighbourhood would know of his suicide attempt and, pointing to a postman who happened to be passing, said 'he'll tell them all about it'. Mr Wrigley appeared not to dwell on these ideas once they occurred to him, and may even have forgotten them shortly afterwards.

Mr Wrigley continued to experience difficulty with his concentration and his memory, for example, he made many mistakes in serially subtracting seven from 100.

Mr Wrigley believed that he was depressed and thought that he would never improve.

An occupational therapy assessment had been performed and Mr Wrigley had begun a limited programme. Many activities were written-off by him as 'no good for a man' but he was drawn to the greenhouse and spoke of his previous skill in the garden. He spoke bitterly of his present 'uselessness', particularly his unemployability, but at the same time berated his employers for not finding him alternative 'light work'. 'If they had, none of this would have happened', he added.

His chest X-ray, full blood count, urea, electrolytes, thyroid function tests and ECG were all normal. Syphilis serology was negative.

He was continuing to take dothiepin, now 150 mg a day, which had been first started in out-patients, and was also taking chlorpromazine 150 mg a day (50 mg in the morning, 100 mg at night).

The most important decision at this stage is whether the present treatment has failed to work and, if so, what are the alternatives. The urgency of this decision will depend on how dangerous to himself Mr Wrigley is considered to be, and this will depend on an accurate reassessment of the severity of his depression.

Reformulation

Diagnosis

All the evidence, including his nearly fatal suicide attempt, confirms that Mr Wrigley is severely depressed. His occasionally abnormally suspicious ideas are consistent with a depressive psychosis but not with a depressive neurosis. No previous episode of mania or evidence of cyclothymic or obsessional personality has emerged on detailed investigation. Although there is now a family history of 'nervous illness' it is not characteristically depressive. There is therefore no evidence of a manic-depressive diathesis and this favours the diagnosis of reactive depressive psychosis.

Mr Wrigley has also developed a weakness of his right hand. This was a spastic paresis associated with sensory loss. It cannot have been present before his suicide attempt because he was then able to hold a thin safety razor blade in his right hand with sufficient strength to sever the tendons of his left wrist.

Two diagnoses need therefore to be considered in formulating Mr Wrigley's management and prognosis:

1. Depressive psychosis.
2. Recent spastic paresis.

Aetiology

Depressive psychosis

There appears to be no backing for Mr Wrigley having a constitutional vulnerability to depression. His family's closeness over the years and his consistently warm accounts of his mother would appear to make it unlikely that Mr Wrigley's upbringing left him with a vulnerability to depression. Although, it must be stressed, very little is known even now, of Mr Wrigley's memories, feelings, or preconceptions which might give a clue about how his early life shaped his present personality and coping abilities. Any theory of a life-long predisposition to depression would anyway have to explain the late onset of Mr Wrigley's illness.

It is notable that Mr Wrigley appears not to have become depressed following his first stroke and his consequent redundancy, but only two weeks after his second stroke which was much less physically disabling. Although it is possible that the two months between strokes was an 'incubation period' during which a depressive reaction was building up as Mr Wrigley's emotional resources became exhausted, it seems more probable that the most important precipitant of Mr Wrigley's depression was the second stroke. This is likely to have had psychological significance, as a further reminder of Mr Wrigley's vulnerability. It is also possible that it had a direct neurobiological effect.

It is likely that Mr Wrigley's unemployment, and an ever increasing spiral of angry and self-critical ruminations linked to it, maintained and aggravated his depression. Although there was a strong undercurrent of anger in his present relationship with his wife, there is no reason to suppose that this was long-standing. Her anger seems an understandable reaction to Mr Wrigley's long, demanding illness and even more, to the unpleasantness of his suicide attempt. His anger remains unexplained but is equally directed at medical and nursing staff as evinced by his 'gallows humour'.

Mr Wrigley's depressive illness appears to have been well-established by the time that his sister died. It is not known whether Mr Wrigley had expected her death, or whether it had contributed to his depression.

The reason that Mr Wrigley made his suicide attempt when he did remains uncertain, and this increases concern about a future attempt. One possible factor is that he might have become more energetic in response to antidepressant treatment, but a similar response did not occur when the same antidepressant was continued after admission.

Spastic paresis

The most likely explanation for this is that an extension of his previous infarct occurred during his episode of haemorrhagic shock.

Further investigation

A great many of the questions previously raised about Mr Wrigley as a person are still unanswered. Historical information has been difficult to gather due to his weak physical condition on admission, to his depression and to his defensive attitudes towards psychiatry and psychiatrists. Enough of a picture has emerged, however, for key items of missing information to be identified and these will be considered, along with other investigations, under the two previous headings plus two 'general' headings.

Depressive psychosis

The nature of Mrs Wrigley's own apparently psychological illness and its relationship to Mr Wrigley's illness needs clarification. Her medical notes should be obtained.

The details of Mr Wrigley's redundancy are unclear. Was he offered alternative employment, redundancy pay or a pension? Who made the decision?

Spastic paresis

The possibility has been raised that Mr Wrigley has suffered further infarction. Although it is unlikely that his cerebral cortex has been affected his cognitive function should be tested after he has recovered from his depressive illness. A further CT scan is probably not indicated.

Suicidal risk

The reasons that Mr Wrigley has for attempting to conceal his illness need to be ascertained. Do his friends and family really only value him when he is the 'life and soul' of the party? Does he have the view that depression is due to 'weakness'? Is he frightened of psychiatric hospitals? Is he ashamed of being a psychiatric patient? Does he think it unmanly to show feelings?

Enquire about the exact circumstances and antecedents of both of Mr Wrigley's suicide attempts. A careful drinking history needs to be taken. Intoxication may 'release' suicidal behaviour and alcohol dependence itself increases the risk of suicide. Are there any traits of Mr Wrigley's character that may have predisposed him to suicide? What is his attitude to it? Does he have any strong religious beliefs which would include beliefs about suicide?

General

There is some information which it is important to obtain from every patient. A drinking history is an example. A lot of this information is missing in Mr Wrigley's case. More needs to be known about his drinking habits, but also about his war service, about his work history, about his sexual history, about any forensic history, and about his financial and domestic circumstances.

There are also one or two features of Mr Wrigley's history, as of any psychiatric history, that stimulate curiosity. Why, for example, is there such a big age gap between the children?

Management

This will also be considered under three headings.

Depression—the acute episode

Mr Wrigley has not responded to over three weeks of treatment with an antidepressant. The course has not been continuous and blood levels of the drug are not available, so Mr Wrigley cannot be considered a non-responder. However, Mr Wrigley's own sense of untreatability, his distress and staff fears for his safety are compelling reasons for changing the treatment. ECT is probably the treatment of choice. It is likely to be at least as effective as an antidepressant and probably quicker. It is not contra-indicated by Mr Wrigley's stroke since this was not a complication of hypertension. Mr Wrigley's tracheotomy was a contra-indication but this has now healed. His physical condition is good. Mr Wrigley is having a modest dose (150 mg) of dothiepin. The alternative to ECT would be to increase this dose until side-effects became apparent or, alternatively, to switch to an antidepressant of known efficacy for which the laboratory could produce blood levels so that drug absorption could be checked.

It is also important to try and reduce Mr Wrigley's self-condemnation and sense of worthlessness. His sense of grievance and the hostility which is associated with his depression have probably contributed to both of these. They can be made more tolerable if they are 'contained' by nursing and medical staff by being listened to, but not argued away. An attempt should also be made to raise Mr Wrigley's self-esteem by providing him with activities which he finds satisfying. In view of his interest in gardening the occupational therapist should be consulted about incorporating this as part of his daily routine.

Mr Wrigley's family should be encouraged to maintain their visits, given the opportunity to express their anxieties, and re-assured that they were not to blame for his illness or for the suicide attempt.

Depression—the long-term

There is a risk that Mr Wrigley's depression will recur if his cir-cumstances to not change. To prevent this an attempt should therefore be made to alter those circumstances that are of aetio-logical importance, for example, by providing Mr Wrigley with some occupation. Re-employment is unlikely in view of his physical state, age and lack of marketable skills, but voluntary work or a day centre are possibilities. The choice would depend on their availability and acceptability to Mr Wrigley. It would be important to suggest an activity that he saw as 'manly'. This would probably be best achieved by some sort of manual work, although Mr Wrigley's weak right hand may restrict the range of suitable activities.

Maintenance antidepressant drugs should probably be given for at least a year. Out-patient follow-up should be offered for at least as long as this and the general practitioner encouraged to refer Mr Wrigley back at an early stage if he should relapse after that. Mr and Mrs Wrigley should also be given the name of a contact person, such as the consultant to contact directly in the event of a relapse.

Brain infarction

Neurological advice should be sought about the use of a long-term antithrombotic agent, such as aspirin. A physiotherapy and later on an occupational therapy programme should be devised to exercise his hand.

Suicide risk

Despite the precautions already discussed, there is a risk that treatment of any relapse may be as delayed or inadequate as present treatment has been. The best safeguard against this is that Mr Wrigley is followed-up by someone who has seen him when he was severely depressed and who has also established a relationship of trust with him.

Prognosis

Mr Wrigley is likely to recover from this episode but, as already mentioned, there is a significant risk of relapse whilst the circumstances that led to his depression continue. Mr Wrigley has also become further disabled as a result of his suicide attempt. He has noticeable scars on his wrists and throat, he has weakness of his right hand and he may have increased cognitive impairment. Should Mr Wrigley relapse, there is a high risk of a further suicide attempt, or successful suicide. The risk is increased by Mr Wrigley's tendency to dismiss the severity of his symptoms, and to mask his misery by superficial jocoseness.

The recurrence of depression will be made more likely if, as is possible, Mr Wrigley considers himself to blame for these disabilities. It would be considerably lessened if suitable occupation could be found for him since Mr Wrigley appears to have been free of depression, and to have coped well with adversity (such as the death of his mother) before his redundancy. Maintenance antidepressant treatment and the establishment of a rapid pathway to psychiatric consultation can also improve the prognosis, as would confidence in the psychiatrist and a greater readiness to consult him in the event of any deterioration.

Further information

Mr Wrigley responded well to six twice-weekly ECT applications. He was discharged to a day hospital three weeks after beginning the course, apparently in normal spirits. His hand, although much improved, was still weak and Mr Wrigley blamed this on the cut on his wrist, saying 'I shouldn't have done it, should I, doctor?' He had a rousing welcome home from his friends but his pleasure at returning to his social club was marred by the discovery that he could no longer join in the sing-songs. His voice since his tracheotomy was not strong enough to hold a sung note.

A case conference was called. Mrs Wrigley's medical notes were obtained, Mr Wrigley's notes studied afresh and Mr Wrigley interviewed again. The history then obtained was as follows.

Mr Wrigley's father, Anthony, probably died of tuberculosis leaving the family in very straitened circumstances. His mother had to get what work she could, which was sometimes only collecting rags for re-sale. The children occasionally went hungry and made use of the Church Army soup kitchen. There had been 4 children: Anthony had died of a brain tumour, Rosy, a sibling who had not been previously mentioned, had died of an infection at the age of 6 months, Flo who had died recently, and Mr Wrigley the youngest. Mr Wrigley's mother appeared to have inspired awe as well as love in Mr Wrigley. Despite the pinched circumstances Mr Wrigley remembered his childhood as being very happy, and his family and their neighbours as being close and supportive. His sister and he continued to live in the same area after his mother died 16 years earlier. However after a few years they were dispersed by an urban renewal scheme and 'something was lost'. After his mother, Mr Wrigley was closest to Flo. Flo had had to stay at home to look after her mother, but after her death Flo married and she and her husband were in the habit of going with the Wrigleys every Sunday to put flowers on his mother's grave.

Mr Wrigley had been a lively boy whose main interest was sport. He played cricket for his school. He had little academic interest and left at 14 to work as a lathe operator.

As the result of a strike three years later he was made redundant and then worked for two years as a plumber's mate until he was called up. Mr Wrigley served as a sapper in Africa and the Far East during the war. He was never promoted and had two periods in a military prison for drunkenness. He resented the pay he received, feeling that he was unable to provide as much for his mother as he wanted. In 1941 his brother was accidentally wounded whilst on active service and was invalided out. He subsequently developed an infection and died. The news reached Mr Wrigley whilst he was in hospital for treatment of dysentery. He requested compassionate leave but this was turned down. He assumed that the accident had caused the infection and felt incensed that the army paid no compensation to his mother. His reaction to the news may have prolonged his stay in hospital although it was not clear whether he was depressed or simply angry.

After the war Mr Wrigley had various jobs in the building trade and then two long periods as a labourer. The second job, with the Water Board paid very well because it involved him in emergency work at night and weekends for which he received 'call-out' rates. Mr Wrigley's last job, with the hospital, came to an end when he had his first stroke. He was on sick leave for about six weeks and was then examined by a doctor acting on behalf of his employers who recommended retirement on medical grounds. Mr Wrigley said that they treated him 'generously'—he received a lump sum and was continuing to have a small pension.

Mr Wrigley went out with his first girlfriend at the age of 16. He had no serious girlfriend until he met his wife at a dance after the war. They married within a year and went to live with his mother. There were often rows about money at the beginning. Mr Wrigley liked to gamble at greyhound races and this prevented them from saving for a house. His mother eventually stepped in with an ultimatum—he either stopped, or 'got out'. Since then he gambled much less but still did so, usually on horse racing. Their son was born a year after they were married. His daughter was 'a mistake'. Neither Mr nor Mrs Wrigley had wanted further children. Mr Wrigley assured the interviewer that he loved her, now, quite as much as his son.

Mrs Wrigley worked as a cleaner until she developed arthritis in 1979 but had not worked since. She had two recent episodes of illness, to be described later. One involved weight loss. Mrs Wrigley was strikingly thin even when this problem had been treated. Her usual weight was 80 lb and her height just under 5 feet. It was difficult to assess how husband and wife felt about each other. Mrs Wrigley found it easier to talk about her exasperation with her husband and his general practitioner and only spoke about her concern in a veiled way, for example, 'I knew that he wasn't right when he'd apologize when I shouted at him instead of shouting back'.

When he was well Mr Wrigley spent three or four weekday evenings at the pub, sometimes with his wife, and regularly went to the British Legion with her on Saturdays. This was the most enjoyable part of the week for him. He would drink three to four pints of bitter at the pub whenever he went out, and the occasional half pint at home on other evenings. They lived in a rented semi-detached three-bedroom house with a pleasant garden. Mr Wrigley enjoyed doing odd jobs in both house and garden, but he was happiest in company. His wife described him as a 'man's man'.

Mr Wrigley's first stroke occurred when he was getting undressed. His right side began to shake and then became stiff. This worsened over several hours and he also developed slurred speech and a droop of the right side of his face. The facial palsy and dysarthria disappeared in a few days but a mild right hemiparesis was still present when he was examined by his general practitioner eight months later, shortly after his second stroke. On this occasion he felt his left arm and leg become cold and weak and then felt himself to be falling to the left. For two weeks following this Mr Wrigley's gait was unsteady. He then developed shaking of his right side which was worse in the morning. Retrospectively this was presumably one of the first symptoms of depression for it was at that time that his family noted a change in his mood. Mr Wrigley was referred to a neurologist for his shakiness who noted early clubbing, minimal unsteadiness and a high erythrocyte sedimentation rate (ESR). He was given a follow-up appointment after which he was discharged.

Mrs Wrigley became ill herself in the meanwhile with what she now referred to as 'a depression'. She described herself as 'doing nothing and eating nothing' and just 'flopping in a chair'. This was attributed at the time to the effect of analgesics.

The situation at home became worse. Mr Wrigley was prescribed benzodiazepines by his general practitioner and was told to stop drinking. This resulted in his not going to the pub and losing contact with his friends. He began to go for long, lonely walks. His sister, Flo, had a stroke and this was found to be due to a cerebral metastasis. Mrs Wrigley kept his sister's illness from her husband for fear that he would think that he had cancer, but when she died he was too 'numb' to feel her death very strongly.

Eight months before admission Mr Wrigley was again referred to a neurologist with 'nervousness, shaking, poor appetite and inability to concentrate'. The neurologist noted that he was markedly depressed and had a classical anxiety tremor. He also noted increased tone, brisk reflexes in all four limbs, more on the left than the right, clonus of his left ankle and a 'probably extensor' left plantar reflex. A diagnosis of 'brain-stem ischaemia/infarction' was made and Mr Wrigley was put on the waiting list for further investigation in hospital.

The Saturday after this, Mr Wrigley suddenly shouted 'I can't stand any more of this' and ran into the kitchen. His sister-in-law ran after him and restrained him from pushing a carving knife into his abdomen. The blade had already penetrated a jumper and shirt and his skin. Mr Wrigley broke down after this, sobbing 'I'm sorry, I'm sorry', as already described.

Mr Wrigley was admitted to hospital three weeks later and his wife was admitted shortly after for investigation of weight loss. Mr Wrigley was noted to have early clubbing, a palpable liver, an abdominal scar, poor co-ordination of his left leg and the spastic signs previously mentioned. The arch aortogram, previously described, was performed at this time. A CT scan was later performed in the out-patient department with the results already described.

Mrs Wrigley was not found to be malabsorbing and her weight loss was attributed to the 'stress of living with her husband'. She saw a psychiatrist who advised her 'to socialize more'. When she returned home, she found her husband's mood had deteriorated further. He roamed the house at night, banged the wall with his fists and avoided contact with family and friends. She tried to persuade her general practitioner to refer him to a psychiatrist but he was reluctant to do so.

The neurologist was also concerned with Mr Wrigley's weight loss and ordered an ultrasound scan of his liver and a barium enema, both of which were found to be normal. Six weeks later the consultant reviewed him in the clinic. He told Mr Wrigley that he had vertebrobasilar insufficiency, that the cause had been found, and that it was under control, but that they had 'drawn a blank' about his weight loss. He recommended referral to a general physician. Mr Wrigley's symptoms did not change markedly between this time and his referral to the psychiatric out-patient department. He did not know what to do with himself and went for long walks or paced the floor. He went very occasionally to the club but did not enjoy it. He avoided meeting people. He slept less and less.

On the day of his suicide attempt Mr Wrigley got up, as usual, at 6.30 a.m. as he would have done if he had been working. He had been awake but lying in bed for some hours before this, but had no particular thoughts of suicide. He went downstairs and heard the men next door and across the road going to work. He suddenly thought 'what's the point?' He had a safety razor blade in his hand and using it he cut repeatedly into his left wrist, thinking 'I might as well finish the job off', he transferred the blade to his left hand and cut his right wrist, and then, with the blade in his right hand, cut his throat. He felt heavy, and then cold, and remembered no more until he was in hospital. From his wife's account it appears that his daughter, who had to get up unusually early, went down a few minutes later and found her father jammed behind the toilet door. Neither she nor her mother had an intimation of his suicide attempt.

The usefulness of a formulation is constrained by the accuracy and completeness of the information obtained. The fresh history brought to light many details of the development of Mr Wrigley's illness, his personality and his background. We consider that a detailed history of this kind, in which there is a narrative quality to the life history and the history of the presenting complaint, is desirable in every patient.

In Mr Wrigley's case, this has resulted in some missing information being obtained, for example, that Mr Wrigley had another sibling who had died, that Tracey was unplanned and that Mr Wrigley had been a heavy gambler. Inaccuracies have also been corrected, for example, the timing of his redundancy in relation to his illness. Even more importantly, a more secure and personal relationship with the psychiatrist has been established.

The events of Mr Wrigley's life now make sense because they are located in a personal context. Mr Wrigley's impulsive and nearly catastrophic suicide attempt can now be seen to be of a piece with his gambling; the anger motivating it can be seen to have been foreshadowed by his anger with the army's refusal of leave to him and compensation to his mother.

It might be argued that in a busy clinic, or in an examination, such detail cannot be obtained. Whilst this is true, we would argue that it is, for this reason, even more important to take detailed histories of in-patients, if necessary spreading the history taking process over the period of their illness and convalescence. Only in this way can an 'ear' for likely developments in a patient's history be acquired. Once a psychiatrist's 'ear' is attuned, much briefer interviews will produce understandable narratives.

The narrative approach is of benefit to the patient, as well as of interest to the psychiatrist. It can throw a light on historical facts which may considerably influence management. If the first psychiatrist who saw Mr Wrigley had appreciated how serious his first impulsive suicide attempt was, that Mr Wrigley had acted on similarly self-destructive impulses before, and how angry he was, he would most likely have seen him the following day and not in two weeks. This might possibly have prevented his suicide attempt, and the consequent distress and disability.

We recommend that the sceptical reader now test this by reconsidering the argument of the initial formulation in the light of the additional information obtained later.

We anticipate that the reader will note how valuable some apparently trivial items of history proved to be in formulating this case. Although the main subject of this book is the skill of organizing and selecting information once it has been obtained in order to formulate a case, we hope that the reader will also become attentive to learning the skill of how this aetiology is involved as the information is being obtained.

We are not, of course, urging the uncritical and unselective amassing of information for its own sake. The goal of information collecting is, after all, to enable the best formulation of treatment and prognosis. However, there is a reciprocal interaction between history-taking and formulation. However impressive the formulation it will be flawed if it is based on an inaccurate or incomplete history and it will be of limited use unless the patient feels that his personal predicament has been understood.

Postscript

Mr Wrigley attended the day hospital for five months. He made many acquaintances in the hospital and greatly enjoyed his work in the garden. The grip in his right hand improved to near normal, and he was eventually able to use it to hold a trowel. However, fine co-ordination and sensation remained impaired.

A place in a local day centre was then found. Mr Wrigley initially attended there part-time and the day hospital part-time, and was then discharged from the hospital to attend the centre full-time. This coincided with an exacerbation of his wife's arthritis, and Mr Wrigley became briefly depressed. However, he recovered without specific treatment, and three months after discharge, was in good spirits and had become established in a small greenhouse at the day centre where he considered himself as having an important role in helping patients less fortunate than himself.

Mr Wrigley continued on a maintenance dose (100 mg) of amitriptyline throughout this period.

3

An overdose—the case of Mary Brown, aged 17

Presenting complaint

The duty psychiatrist was asked to see Mary who had been admitted to the observation ward following an overdose of about 40 aspirins two days previously. This was described in the notes as an 'impulsive overdose' which followed a series of rows with her boyfriend. When she saw the psychiatrist, Mary said that she felt 'very confused' about the situation she was in and wanted to 'hear someone else's point of view'. She then gave the following account of the circumstances surrounding her overdose.

It had followed one of her frequent rows with Cyril, her boyfriend. They had gone out for a walk and returned to his house to have sexual intercourse. After this, he began to question her about her previous boyfriends and to complain that he had no confidence in her faithfulness. This developed into an argument and she started to challenge him about his previous girlfriends. He then 'smacked me around the face and walked out of the room'. She said that she then felt 'frustrated and helpless' and picked up a bottle of aspirins which she kept under her pillow to treat headaches. She took all the aspirins in the bottle (about 40) because she 'just wanted to get out of this awful situation'. At that moment she believed she would have taken even more tablets if they had been available, although she generally had considerable difficulty swallowing even one.

About half an hour later she began to feel sick and generally unwell. She then panicked and ran out to tell Cyril, who was downstairs. He tried to make her vomit by putting his fingers down her throat, but this failed and he called an ambulance which took her to the casualty department. After her stomach was washed out, Cyril continued to berate her about her previous affairs and she then felt very relieved to be admitted to hospital.

Family history

Her adoptive mother was 55 and managed a hairdressing salon.
Mary said that she 'alternated between loving and hating her'.
She generally found it easy to discuss problems with her. However, her mother strongly disapproved of Cyril and they therefore avoided talking about him. Her adoptive father was 55 and
managed an advertising agency. His physical health had deteriorated over the last 18 months during which time he had
suffered several minor strokes. According to Mary, this meant
that he was unable to maintain responsibility for his business and
his partners were therefore forced to take over more of its active
management. Apparently, he was unaware of this. She said that
they got on 'quite well', but she found him difficult to talk to
because he always saw things in 'black and white' terms.

She had a 19-year-old adoptive brother, John, and described
their relationship as 'wonderful'. He was extremely intelligent
and did well at school. She said that her parents approved of his
circle of friends and she thought that he was allowed far more
freedom than her. Her adoptive mother had had a stillbirth
before she and John were adopted.

Mary said she was told nothing about her natural mother, but
from conversations she had overheard she believed that she was
a French refugee who had been evacuated to England and
became pregnant after an affair with a married English soldier.
When asked directly she said that she bore little resemblance to
either of her adoptive parents, although she did resemble John.

Personal history

Mary was born in Wales and was adopted within a few months of
her birth. She was brought up in Liverpool and remembered her
childhood as an 'extremely happy one' and believed that her
knowing about her adoption never spoiled her relationship with
her parents. She felt grateful to them for being so 'honest' and
'open' about this because it made their relationship more 'adult'.
As far as she was concerned, the fact that she was physically dis-
similar to both her parents had never been a problem. The family
were always very comfortably off. She had nice clothes, enjoy-

able holidays (frequently taken abroad), and they lived in a large comfortable house.

She attended a local school from the age of four, which she described as 'enjoyable' and where she made many friends. Initially, she did quite well at school. However, as she became older she became increasingly uninterested in her school work and was often told off by her teachers for talking in class. Eventually, she came to dislike school, but she also said 'I do not think I would have liked any school I would have attended'. When she was 16 she passed three GCE O levels, but believed that she should have passed all the six subjects that she had taken. Although she had many friends at school most of them lived a considerable distance away from her and she did not maintain contact with them outside school hours. On occasions, she played truant with friends, but this was never discovered and she said that she never came into serious conflict with the school staff.

After she took her O levels she left school and found herself a job as a beauty consultant, which she kept for six weeks. She got on badly with her supervisor and because of this she left to join a beauty consultant agency in a temporary capacity. However, there was insufficient work available for her and she left this job after four months. Following several months of unemployment she found herself another job as a receptionist for a voluntary organization which she also left after two weeks because she found it 'boring'. For the last 15 months she had been unemployed.

Her menarche occurred when she was 12. She said that she did not start going out with boys until she was 15, at which time she had her first sexual relationship. This took place while she was on holiday abroad with her parents and it was with a man 25 years older than herself. Following this she had numerous, brief sexual relationships which she described as 'very enjoyable'. Six months previously she had met her current boyfriend, Cyril, at a party given by some friends of her brother. She said that she had no other boyfriends since. Cyril was 20 years old, black, unemployed, and came from a large, working-class family. Her parents completely disapproved of this relationship, mainly because of Cyril's colour. This led to frequent rows at home and she began to spend increasingly less time at home and more time with Cyril. Eventually, her mother told her to leave home and she found herself a flat.

For the last three months she had lived with Cyril and his family in their house. She described his family as 'extremely supportive and friendly, but not pushy'. Since they were both unemployed, they spent practically all their time together and had frequent sexual intercourse, which she enjoyed. However Cyril continually brought up details of her previous relationships and continued to criticize her for these. On several occasions he physically assaulted her, but she said that she was never seriously hurt by him and as far as she was concerned their relationship recovered rapidly following these arguments. She said that she had no other friends apart from Cyril and his family. These rows became increasingly frequent and she began to feel very hurt and upset about Cyril's continual demand that she promise to be faithful. It was following one of these arguments that she took her overdose.

Past medical history

Six months previously, Mary was treated for a gonococcal infection which she said she had contracted from Cyril.

Two months previously, she suffered a severe attack of herpes genitalis, which had only just cleared up.

She had suffered no other serious medical illness but did describe recurrent attacks of 'headaches'. She described these as 'tightness around my head', which often followed her arguments with Cyril and were relieved by taking aspirins.

Past psychiatric history

Mary gave no history of any previous psychiatric illness.

Previous personality

Mary described herself as always having been a friendly, outgoing person and she did not think she had changed.

Mental state examination

Appearance and general behaviour

Mary was an overweight, but attractive red-head, who smiled frequently during the interview and conveyed a sense of flirtatiousness. She was relaxed and self-composed and had clearly taken some care about her appearance, since she wore smart clothes and was effectively made up.

Talk

She spoke clearly and fluently.

Mood

Although Mary looked quite miserable when she discussed her relationship with Cyril, this was not sustained. Most of the time she appeared reasonably cheerful and she smiled frequently. She said that she had no concerns about her physical health and was not particularly bothered by her headaches. She did not give the impression of being concerned about her femininity. Although she frequently said that she felt 'guilty' about her promiscuity and her current relationship with her family, she did not convey this feeling with any intensity. She described her current difficulties as 'unresolvable', but presented this as an intriguing state of affairs rather than a problem which overwhelmed her. She said that she never thought of taking an overdose before and 'certainly never' made any such threats to Cyril. She also said that she had no intention of killing herself at the time, but added 'when you are feeling upset you don't care . . .'. When asked directly she agreed that she had felt angry, but mainly upset. Following the overdose she became very frightened that she might die and was relieved to have obtained such speedy assistance. On reflection, she felt that it was 'a very silly thing to have done', but felt that it had at least forced a confrontation between Cyril and herself and that this would be useful. However, she did not think that this would become a means of getting her own way in the future and she said she would never take an overdose again.

Thought content

Mary talked a great deal about her intense feelings for Cyril. She said that she found him physically attractive and sexually satisfying and felt that he often showed considerable sympathy for the difficulties she experienced with her family. She also found his family relaxed, warm, and friendly and felt that they had accepted and welcomed her. On the other hand, she found his continual cross-questioning about her previous relationships exhausting and frustrating and she was beginning to feel at a loss as to how she would be able to reassure him satisfactorily about the future. She then said 'I often feel I would be unable to reassure myself about this too'. At the same time, she felt that Cyril was also being very unreasonable to insist on her faithfulness when he was continuing to be promiscuous. As far as she was concerned she loved him, but 'I can't live with him and I can't live without him'.

She frequently referred to herself as a 'slag' and said that she understood why Cyril mistrusted her and why he continually needed to seek reassurance. On the other hand, she now believed that his was 'all behind me' and felt frustrated at having to continually go over the past. She said that she felt certain she had changed and was fed up with being reminded about her previous relationships. When asked directly about these relationships she said that she had enjoyed the sexual side, but never really became emotionally involved with anyone before Cyril.

Mary expressed considerable curiosity about her natural mother and said that she hoped to find out more about her. She described how she had contacted Somerset House to obtain a copy of her birth certificate but was informed that this would not be available to her until she reached 18. She also began to worry that her adoptive mother would get upset if she found out about her enquiry.

Mary frequently described how concerned she felt about the situation at home. She felt that looking after her adoptive father was increasingly difficult and that she should have spent more time at home helping. She said that she felt irresponsible for leaving her parents to sort out these problems themselves and giving them extra worries about herself. However, she also said that there was no practical help she could offer at home anyway.

When Mary described her relationship with her family and her early upbringing, it was noticeable how much effort she put into pointing out her appreciation for their care and concern. She also pointed out how she understood the difficulties they might have faced in bringing her up. On the other hand, she was never specific about these 'difficulties' and when asked directly about them she rejected the suggestion that they might have anything to do with her having been adopted.

She made it clear on several occasions that she did not want anyone in her family to be informed of her current situation.

Abnormal beliefs and interpretation of events

None were elicited.

Abnormal experiences

None were elicited.

Cognitive state

This was not formally tested, but Mary appeared well orientated in time and space and of above average intelligence.

Appraisal of illness

Mary did not think that she was suffering from a psychiatric illness, but saw her problems resulting from her relationship with Cyril. She did not think her overdose was a serious suicide attempt, but a way of getting herself out of an awkward situation. She thought that having taken the overdose, things would probably settle down.

Physical examination

A thorough physical examination had been performed by the physician and nothing abnormal had been found. Investigations had shown that her serum salicylate level never reached a dangerous level and dropped to zero by the time she was examined by the psychiatrist.

Ward observations

The nurses described Mary as a 'normal, cheerful girl' who talked freely and openly with them and the other patients on the ward. She was helping the elderly ladies there, by making cups of tea. She never cried and appeared to be sleeping and eating well.

Her boyfriend had turned up on two occasions and they seemed to get on quite amicably.

Summary

Mary Brown is a 17-year-old adopted white girl who has taken an overdose following an argument with her black boyfriend.

Young, female patients who have taken an overdose are unlikely either to have a persistent psychiatric disorder or to attend any follow-up appointment. As a result of this and other pressures, such as the general work-load, when psychiatrists examine such patients they set out to exclude a serious psychiatric disorder and avoid making management plans based upon a detailed evaluation of the individual's requirements. Although this may be justified on the grounds of expediency it is not an approach that can generally be recommended and in this case these issues will be considered.

Formulation

Diagnosis

Some of Mary's symptoms could be seen as manifestations of a depressive illness. On several occasions she said how 'guilty' she felt about her previous sexual promiscuity and neglecting her family. She also denigrated herself by referring to herself as a 'slag'. However, these feelings were not conveyed with a morbid intensity and did not contain a hopeless quality. In fact, she appeared to accept them as a rather temporary state of affairs for which she did not feel totally responsible. Her feeling that she had no contribution to make to her family's welfare seemed to be less important than her relationship with Cyril. However, although she regretted her past promiscuity she also said that she wanted Cyril to stop pestering her about it. Essentially, her feelings of 'guilt' appeared to reflect a realistic discomfort with her current circumstances and a wish for the situation to be changed, rather than an unremitting, deep discontent with herself, over which she had not control.

No other features were found that might support a diagnosis of depression. She appeared cheerful, described no alteration in her sleep pattern, and did not report any changes in her mood. However, the information available does suggest that she had serious problems in establishing and maintaining interpersonal relationships. She has never had any long-standing, close friendship or childhood friend. Although her explanation for this was that she lived too far away from school, this does not explain why she was unable to make friends closer to her home. Her main relationships were with men, were brief and seem to have been based solely on sexual attraction. Her longest sustained relationship, with Cyril, had the additional disturbing feature of frequent rows, occasionally developing into physical fights.

Her school record suggested that she under-achieved and there is a suspicion that she had problems with her teachers as well as with her peers. The possibility that she had problems with authority is reinforced by her work record. According to her she had less difficulty obtaining employment than in holding down a job for any length of time. Although she gave 'boredom' as her reason for leaving, on at least one occasion she admitted to having had difficulties with her employer.

Finally, although she evaded going into detail, she conveyed the impression that she had long-standing problems with her family. She had considerable conflict with them over Cyril and was forced to leave home on account of this. She implied that she found her brother more favoured by her parents, even though she said that her relationship with him was 'wonderful'. Furthermore, the fact that she so strenuously attempted to understand why her parents might have had problems with her supports the belief that there were difficulties. This is reinforced by the importance she placed upon Cyril's family's attitude towards her, which she described as 'warm and caring'. However, she steadfastly resisted being explicit about these issues.

Examination of her mental state also revealed several noteworthy features. In particular, she maintained a cheerful, relaxed posture in spite of her insistence that she was in an awful situation from which she felt she could never escape. This suggests quite marked dissociation of affect. She also appeared to obtain considerable gratification from discussing her problems while expressing the belief that she would have to sort them out herself. Finally, the psychiatrist was struck not only by her 'charming' manner (which appears inconsistent with the situation she was describing) but by the element of flirtatiousness in her behaviour. One effect of this was that he did not pursue her statements thoroughly. For example, he did not clarify whether the aspirins she kept under her pillow for 'headaches' reflected a long-standing preoccupation with self-harm.

In summary, Mary had few close interpersonal relationships and the relationships she did have were coloured by shallowness of affect and difficulty in accepting control from authority. She also showed possible dissociation of affect and a seeming gratification from being in impossible situations. Furthermore, she presented herself in a way that made it very difficult to challenge or clarify important issues which emerged. Many of these characteristics can be observed at some time in most people, particularly when they are placed under stress. However, in Mary's case they were all present together and significantly coloured her behaviour, particularly in the context of her recent overdose.

These features are compatible with a diagnosis of either an hysterical personality disorder or an acute adjustment reaction. The possibility of Mary having an hysterical personality disorder is supported by the suggestion that these elements have coloured Mary's relationships since childhood and are now an established part of her character structure. However, it is also possible that although these elements were present, they contributed less significantly to her character and have been exaggerated by the current, severe stresses she described. If the emphasis is placed upon the degree of stress rather than personality, then the diagnosis of acute adjustment reaction becomes more likely.

The distinction between these diagnoses is not always clear-cut and frequently depends upon evaluation of outcome. Furthermore, the only available evidence has been obtained from Mary and it requires independent confirmation to support one of these diagnoses. Suspicion remains however, that the disturbances described are sufficiently ingrained to be considered a manifestation of an hysterical personality disorder.

Aetiology

Mary has recently been subjected to several stresses which could have contributed to her overdose. Her adoptive father is becoming physically and intellectually incapacitated as a result of several 'strokes'. This deterioration and the risk of further, possibly fatal 'strokes' would make Mary very vulnerable to an emotional disturbance. Although the time relationship between Mary's disorder and her adoptive father's illness has not been established, her account suggests that this deterioration may also have been associated with her leaving home.

Mary also described two episodes of venereal disease. These might not only have been upsetting experiences, but the fact that herpes genitalis can be very painful could also have made it an additional provocative factor.

Mary's conflictual relationship with Cyril is also likely to have made her vulnerable to taking an overdose and their recent row seems to have been the most immediate trigger. However, she has never taken an overdose before in spite of many previous fights with him and it is unclear whether this row differed in some way from the others or whether it was the last of an accumulation of stresses.

Mary has also talked openly about her wish to trace her natural mother and she will soon be entitled to do this. Anxieties associated with this possibility may also have contributed to her stress at this time.

Although these factors explain why Mary was at risk of taking an overdose at this particular time, she also appears to have an underlying personality disorder which would make her particularly vulnerable. It would not have been surprising if Mary's adoption had affected her personality development and her relationships with her adoptive family. A notable feature in Mary's case is the considerable effort she puts into rejecting this possibility. She insisted that 'it has never been a problem'. She frequently said how 'grateful' she felt to them for the fact that they were always so 'open' about her adoption. She said that she appreciated this and valued their care and attention, although she clearly felt that they favoured her brother.

It is possible that Mary's adoption was not as smooth as she described. Her account, particularly with its inconsistencies, might reflect that she did not always feel comfortable or accepted or loved within her adoptive family and was uncertain about her true identity. This view is reinforced by the importance Mary invested in her relationship with Cyril and his family.

Mary's romanticized account of her natural mother and the

stereotype description she gave of her adoptive parents suggests that she has not developed a clear sense of who she is. This mixture of romanticism with a lack of objectivity and reality coloured her description of her relationship with Cyril. She said 'I can't live with him and I can't live without him'.

The uncertainty about her background and her difficulty in believing that she was accepted by her adoptive family would have made it difficult for her to find an acceptable model with whom to identify during her development. This would then have made it difficult for her to develop strong internal resources which would help her cope with external stresses. These factors would also account for the fact that Mary seemed to dissociate her feelings and present a rather novelettish account of her history, which might seem to her to be more attractive than the uncertainty which really exists.

The factors in Mary's personality which made her vulnerable to stress may also have made her more liable to encounter situations in which she is likely to be stressed. An example of this was her conflictual relationship with Cyril. She seems to have managed her own insecurity by living with someone who is equally insecure. The fact that Cyril was black, unemployed, and extremely jealous was balanced by his apparent capacity to demonstrate affection and the fact that he came from a family she perceived as warm and close.

Further investigations

Although psychiatrists may make decisions based upon one interview, this is generally an unsatisfactory course of action to follow and it is important to try to obtain information from independent sources. One reason for this in Mary's case is that she could be lying. If this were so it would alter both the diagnostic and aetiological possiblities. Even if Mary were not lying, she could be distorting the facts considerably. The fact that her story is quite melodramatic reinforces this possiblity.

The most obvious sources of information are Mary's adoptive parents and Cyril. Her adoptive family should be asked to describe her early development, in particular whether she has always been a disobedient child who was difficult to control. They could confirm whether such traits affected her schooling and resulted in poor school reports or truancy and if they thought this also contributed to her poor work record. They could also give more information concerning her adoption and how much of this was discussed with Mary. The details of Mary's adoptive father's illness should also be clarified, as should the impact of Mary's relationship with Cyril upon her family. An account should be obtained of her general relationships with a peer group and any suspicion that Mary abused drugs.

Cyril could also give his account of their relationship. In particular he could describe their rows in more detail and he could report whether Mary has threatened to take an overdose in the past, or whether he was surprised by this action. It would also be useful to know the extent to which Mary was welcomed by his family.

While attempting to verify these details, the psychiatrist should also attempt to evaluate Mary's relationships with the informants. In particular, it might become apparent whether certain issues would benefit from joint counselling which would be influenced by whether Mary intended to return home or to carry on living with Cyril. More complicated factors like her motivation for joint counselling could also be assessed. For these reasons joint interviews should be encouraged.

Management

The major role of management is to reduce the risk that Mary will take further, serious overdoses when she is placed under stress. This might be achieved by exploring ways in which she can be helped to become less dangerous and more appropriate ways of communicating her distress or by looking for particular areas of stress which might be effectively reduced. All of these approaches can be included within a counselling programme which could be undertaken either individually or jointly with Mary's family and/or with Cyril. In this way particular areas of difficulty could be focused on, such as her rows with Cyril, her difficulty coping with her father's illness, or possible problems concerning her adoption. These alternatives all require her co-operation over an extended period of time and it is therefore necessary to encourage her to attend the out-patient department for follow-up and for her relatives and Cyril to be interviewed.

In order to achieve this the psychiatrist will need to emphasize that he considers her situation to be serious, but that he thinks there are several ways in which he might be able to help her. It would probably also be helpful if he points out straight away to Mary that he does not think she has a psychiatric illness and that she will need to be involved in the decisions regarding further treatment.

Prognosis

Any prediction about the outcome of this episode, in particular Mary's risk of taking another overdose, can only be offered in the uncertainty that surrounds much of the information she has provided. Further details of her personality development, background, and current situation may well affect the prognosis.

In spite of these reservations, most of the available information suggests that Mary has a high risk of further self-harm. She seems to have a personality which makes her vulnerable to stress, she has few friends, lacks internal resources and there is a suspicion that she has had difficulties with authority for some time. Furthermore, she is currently unemployed and has had numerous short-term relationships, both of which increase her vulnerability. Finally, her current relationship with Cyril involves a considerable amount of conflict and has already led to this admission. If she returns to this situation it seems likely that the stresses will continue.

Brief Formulation

Miss Brown is a 17-year-old single white girl who has taken an overdose following an argument with her boyfriend. This appears to have been the latest in a series of rows mainly about her previous sexual activity, which have punctuated their relationship. On examination, she shows no features of a psychiatric illness, rationalizes her problems, is quite flirtatious and exhibits some dissociation of affect.

Diagnosis

The most likely diagnosis is an hysterical personality disorder. It is less likely that this is an acute adjustment reaction and there is no evidence to suggest that she has a depressive illness.

Aetiology

The fact that she was adopted has probably caused considerable problems of identification and her approaching birthday means that she may be anxious about discovering the facts concerning her natural mother. She appears to have had long-standing difficulties with authority figures and has recently been told to leave home because of her relationship with her boyfriend. Her personality seems to have made her vulnerable to developing conflictual relationships, such as the one she has with her boyfriend. She is also currently unemployed and recently suffered two episodes of venereal disease, the second being of a particularly painful type. Finally her adoptive father appears to be seriously unwell and this may be causing considerable distress.

Further investigations

Objective accounts of both Mary's upbringing and her recent behaviour need to be obtained from her adoptive family and from her boyfriend. Her general practitioner could also provide some of this information.

Management

This should be directed towards reducing further episodes of self harm and she should therefore be encouraged to attend the outpatient department, either alone or with her family and/or boyfriend.

Prognosis

There is a significant likelihood of further overdose, particulary if she chooses to return to a conflictual situation and refuses the offer of further help.

Further information

The psychiatrist who assessed Mary accepted her account. He formed the opinion that she had a personality disorder and had taken her overdose as a response to her argument with Cyril. He asked to speak to Cyril and her family, but she refused to let him. He then suggested that she attend the out-patients department in order to discuss her problems further, but she declined this offer as well.

He then decided not to pressurize her any further because he thought she was determined not to attend for follow-up. He considered it more useful to acknowledge this and to suggest that if she were to change her mind he would be pleased to see her again. He also pointed out that she could contact her general practitioner if she felt a further crisis was developing and that this would be a better way of communicating her distress, than to acquire the habit of taking overdoses. Mary smiled and said 'I have to sort out my problems for myself'. She said she had no intention of taking another overdose, but agreed to contact the psychiatrist if she changed her mind.

Following her discharge from hospital, the psychiatrist contacted her general practitioner, who had known Mary and her family for many years. The physician gave the following account of her background.

Mary had been adopted within a week or two of her birth. The adoption was arrange privately by the senior partner of the practice, who knew both Mary's natural mother and her adoptive family. Her current general practitioner had never met Mary's mother but knew that she came from a family with an infamous reputation within the local community. They lived in an extremely deprived area and had a reputation for continual conflict with the police over petty theft and alcoholism. Even within the local community they were considered particularly difficult and made more use of the social services department than other needy families. Mary's general practitioner remarked spontaneously upon the contrast between Mary's natural mother and her adoptive parents' social backgrounds. He confirmed that her adoptive parents were both successful, professional people, that Mr Brown was suffering from a severe pre-senile dementia and that he was now totally incapable of running his business independently. As a result of this, the business was being wound down and this was producing considerable strain—both emotional and financial—for his wife.

Mary had been difficult from a very early age. As a small child her parents frequently complained about her naughtiness, which contrasted markedly with the docility of her adoptive brother. The general practitioner's daughter had attended the same private school as Mary, where she acquired a reputation for being difficult and associated with a group of girls who were demarcated by their persistent disobedience and lack of academic success. He also believed that there was an episode when she was involved in petty theft, but that the matter was hushed up by her family.

He said that she frequently ran away from home and confirmed that three months ago she had left home to live with a West Indian boy, who was unknown to him.

The general practitioner was not surprised that Mary had taken an overdose in view of the problems he noted over the years in her relationships with her family and others.

The psychiatrist also contacted the Registrar for Births and Deaths to clarify the process whereby adoptive children are able to trace their natural parents. This broadly confirmed the account Mary gave, in that adopted children without birth certificates are only able to obtain the appropriate records after they have reached 18 years of age. The leaflet that the psychiatrist received about this devoted a considerable amount of space to explain the importance of counselling for children who pursued this aim.

Mary's current social situation has been broadly confirmed, whereas the details of her adoptive family and previous personality are not wholly unsuspected. The reader should consider whether the psychiatrist would have been able to 'engage' her more successfully if he had obtained this information earlier.

Reformulation

Diagnosis

The additional information makes much clearer the long-standing nature of Mary's problems. She has always been a 'diffi-

cult' child for her adoptive parents as well as for her school-
teachers. There is also a suggestion that she has previously
displayed antisocial tendencies, such as her possible involement
in theft. However, it is the fact that her behavioural problems
have been present from a very early age and seem to have
become established aspects of her personality that make the
diagnosis of hysterical personality disorder much clearer.

Aetiology

The fact that Mary was adopted also takes on increasing significance. It suggests how her personality development may have
been affected, as well as why she has presented at this time.

It may appear strange that her personality resembled her
natural mother's so closely in contrast with that of her adoptive
parents. One possible explanation for this is that she was far
more aware of her mother's character than she revealed and in
some way identified with her. This awareness need not necessarily have been fully conscious and it is possible that her parents
knew her natural mother's background and communicated this to
her, in spite of efforts to protect her from this knowledge. It is
also possible that Mary inherited some personality characteristics from her mother. However, although it is possible that
some specific aspects of her personality may have been transmitted by these means, it is difficult to explain such a complicated mixture of traits of Mary demonstrates.

As far as the timing of Mary's overdose is concerned the
approach of her eighteenth birthday means that she is now in a
position to trace her natural mother. Given the clearer picture of
her natural mother's background, the contrast between this and
her stated expectation would be confronted, and would result in
considerable and understandable distress.

Finally, the general practitioner has also confirmed that Mary's
adoptive father is becoming increasingly incapacitated by a pre-
senile dementia, which is causing considerable distress for his
family. This stress appears to have been related to Mary leaving
home as well as her recent overdose.

Further investigations

It would be useful to know how aware Mary's adoptive family were of her natural mother's personality and background and the extent to which this had been overtly or covertly transmitted to Mary.

Management

The additional information suggests that if any further action can be taken it should be for Mary to obtain specific counselling focusing on two issues. First, the problems surrounding her adoptive father's current illness, and secondly, the problems concerning her natural mother. The main difficulty with this is that Mary has decided not to see the psychiatrist again and therefore the possibility of writing to her offering such a course of action should be considered.

It seems unlikely, given her previous history and the evidence from the interview, that she will accept such a course of action. On the other hand, although it may be more expedient not to contact her, it might be more productive to give her the opportunity of refusing a specific offer of help. An alternative to contacting her directly would be to inform the general practitioner who could refer her back later.

Prognosis

Mary remains at a high risk of taking further overdoses, whether she succeeds in tracing her mother or not. Her personality appears to be well-established and she has shown considerable resistance to accepting offers of help.

Postscript

The psychiatrist decided not to contact Mary again. However, he did contact her general practitioner six months later and established that neither he nor the hospital had received any information about subsequent overdoses.

4

An eating disorder—the case of Jane Morgan, aged 17

Presenting complaint

Jane Morgan was a 17-year-old girl referred by her general practitioner to the psychiatric out-patient department because of severe weight loss and her dread of becoming fat.

One year earlier she had begun to diet with a group of girl-friends at the college she was attending. She weighed 8½ st (54 kg) then and was 5 ft 4 in tall. Jane's initial aim was to lose 'about half a stone' (3 kg) and she was particularly keen to take some fat off her thighs. Within a few weeks the other girls started to give up their diet whereas Jane found that she was able to persist in eating less. She felt proud of this and decided to see how much more weight she could lose. Over the next six months she dropped to 6 st 13 lb (44 kg). She then started eating even less and stopped her mother from cooking an evening meal for her. At this time she was eating food amounting to about 600 calories per day with a typical evening meal being three to four crispbreads spread thinly with cucumber spread. Occasionally she would eat fish but only if it was grilled. As well as this she exercised vigorously in her room every evening.

Jane went on holiday with her mother to Spain in the summer when she weighed 6 st 6 lb (41 kg). There she walked whenever possible and with the rest of the party contracted a gastrointestinal disorder which gave her diarrhoea. She was pleased about this and deliberately ate a lot of fruit to make it worse. It helped her to lose more weight and on her return from holidays she weighed 6 st (38 kg). Despite this she insisted on playing lacrosse with her club.

When her mother offered her food she became angry and stormed out of the room. When she did eat at home she frequently did so standing up and would immediately go out for a long walk. At this time Jane weighed herself six times every day and felt relieved when she noted a further loss of weight.

Two months before presentation to the psychiatric clinic, her mother finally coaxed Jane into going to see the family doctor. She weighed 5 st 9 lb (36 kg) and was now too exhausted to play lacrosse. The doctor, however, was unable to persuade her to eat more and finally referred her to the psychiatrist.

During the last few months Jane had also become extremely fastidious about housework. She was almost continually tidying up and putting things away. She took over nearly all of the cooking and prepared rich and elaborate dishes which she pressured her mother into consuming. She was preoccupied with the need not to waste food. She felt very active and alert and woke at 5 a.m. every day.

One month before her visit to the clinic her father returned from Los Angeles because of his concern about her condition. Her parents insisted that she stop work at this time.

It had been a struggle to get Jane to the clinic but she finally relented because 'my mother looked so miserable'.

Family history

Jane's parents separated when she was 18 months old and they divorced subsequently. Her father, aged 52, was an executive for an oil company and he now lived in Los Angeles. Jane described him as a 'fitness fanatic' who was always concerned about 'healthy living'. He was in the habit of jogging three to four miles every day and he had a particular loathing for 'fat' people. He was a man who read extensively and who always liked to be right in an argument. Everyone regarded him as a 'born leader' and he was energetic in pursuing his aims. Despite the divorce, Mr Morgan maintained regular contact with his family and visited them every year usually bringing expensive presents for the children. Jane remembered that he always seemed to like having attractive women around him.

Jane's mother was 47 and until recently had been a housewife, financially supported by her ex-husband. She had, six months previously, become a registered child minder. Jane described her mother as someone who 'feels deeply but can't express her feelings to others'. In many respects she was the opposite of her father, seeming to be unsure about herself and finding it difficult to make decisions. She was a deeply religious woman and her social activities were restricted to the church. Her appearance was of little concern to her and despite being a little overweight, she had never attempted to diet.

Jane did not know why her parents had separated. She believed, however, that her mother still missed her father and she had never shown any interest in other men. She suspected that her father had many girlfriends. She said she had a good relationship with both of her parents and felt particularly close to her mother and they spent much time together. She often felt intimidated by her father's overbearing personality but felt excited when she knew he was due to visit.

Jane had one sister, Rachel, aged 21, who was a secretary and had left her mother's home to join her father in the United States six months earlier. Since the age of 18 she had had 'itchy feet' and always wanted to travel. She had been to visit her father when he was stationed in New York and later in Los Angeles. She expressed dissatisfaction with home and complained that her mother and Jane were dull, wishing only to go to Church. Jane described Rachel as 'practically like father—intelligent and outspoken'. The two sisters used to fight 'like cat and dog' when children but the relationship had improved recently. Rachel was a constant dieter. When she was 18 she had lost quite a lot of weight but had quickly put it on again. Jane had often teased her about her diets in the past.

There was no family history of psychiatric or physical illness.

Personal history

Jane was born in Dallas, Texas while her father was working for a company there. Her parents had lived there for six years having emigrated from England. In the first two years of Jane's life, her parents moved frequently, four times in the space of one year. When she was 18 months old her parents separated and for the next five years her father visited most Saturdays.

Despite her parents' problems, Jane described her early childhood as a happy one. She showed no behavioural problems.

When she was seven years old, her mother brought her two

daughters back to England while her father remained in the United States. Jane remembered the return as a 'great adventure'. They lived with her grandmother for about a year and then moved into the house in which Jane and her mother still live.

Jane enjoyed junior school, both in the United States and later in England. She made friends easily and was popular on her return because of the novelty of her American accent. She said she was not very bright at school and found it difficult to remember what she should have learnt. However, she excelled at sports and she sang in the school choir. She left school at 16, with five CSEs but having failed two O levels. She said she disliked it as she had to travel long distances to get there.

Eventually she passed two O levels in English and Religious Knowledge and in addition did a typing course. Her school experiences had made her feel 'definitely not academic'.

Immediately after leaving college Jane obtained a job as a secretary in a small frozen food firm and she had worked there for a year up to the time of her presentation to hospital. She said she loved the work because it was varied and because the people were very kind to her. They had shown a lot of concern about her thinness but she was not irritated by this. Her boss had told her father that he would keep the job open because she was a 'good little worker'.

Jane had her menarche at 15 years of age. This was later than her friends who had teased her for being a 'baby'. Her periods were regular until eight months previously, stopping when she weighed 7 st 1 lb (45 kg).

Jane said she was not interested in boys. For her and her best friend, 'lacrosse was our life'. Her friend, however, became engaged nine months previously and they now rarely saw each other. Jane said that her mother always put a 'damper' on her and boys. 'I was always Mum's girl'. Despite being asked out often at college she had never had a boyfriend. She said that she was taught at church that sex was sinful and she disliked the idea of being fondled by boys. She also said that she did not think she could get a steady boyfriend because she was not 'perfection'. She was scared of boys hurting her. When asked if she was sexually attracted to girls she indicated that this was a disgusting suggestion.

Past medical history

Jane had suffered no serious illness in the past. However, when she was 15 she had a cosmetic operation to remove a birth mark on her forehead, having been very sensitive about this 'deformity' for some years. The results was not totally satisfactory to her and she ensured that her forehead was always covered by her hair.

Previous personality

Jane had always been a 'sports fanatic'. She had been in many school teams and had represented her county at lacrosse. She was also a very strong squash player. Recently she had lacked the energy to play. She was also very musical and had played the piano and recorder and was a good singer.

She found it easy to make friends and was generally a cheerful and popular girl with a sense of humour which was often complimented by others.

She had always been conscientious in her work and she tended to live an orderly life. She liked fixed routines and felt uneasy if these were disturbed.

She attended church regularly with her mother but, although she was religious, she was not as devoted as her mother. She did not drink alcohol and had never experimented with any illicit drugs.

Mental state examination

Appearance and general behaviour

Jane was a blonde, wide-eyed, alert, emaciated girl who would obviously have been very attractive if she were not so thin. During the initial part of the interview she responded sullenly to questions but she brightened up as it progressed. She made it clear that she was only there under duress and that she was only co-operating because of her parents' wishes—'I know I am worrying my parents half to death'.

Talk

Jane gave a very articulate account of herself.

Mood

Jane said that she had been feeling depressed over the previous three months. She attributed this to her mother's 'unreasonable fussiness' about her eating. On occasions she had been tearful but denied any feelings of hopelessness about the future. 'If people would only leave me alone everything would be OK'. She expressed some guilt about the effect she had on her mother but the worst guilt was when she ate 'too much'. Her social life was now very poor—'I don't feel like going out—if people ring I get Mum to answer and make up excuses. I just feel like hiding in a corner'. She had lost interest in singing in the church choir—'I don't have the energy to sing any more'. Jane had difficulty with her sleep and woke at 5 a.m. 'Sometimes it hurts when I roll over in bed'. She said, however, that she felt bright and active in the morning. Jane said that she had never thought life was not worth living and had never contemplated suicide. She admitted that sometimes she got 'confused'—'I get angry with myself and say what am I playing at? But then I decide that I can cope all right'. Since her father's return she had felt better—'We've had a good sing-song together'.

Although Jane denied any anxieties other than those surrounding eating, she said that she was somewhat troubled by her 'obsession with housework and order'. 'If something has been moved, I have to get up and put it back in its right place—or if something has been messed up, I have to clean it right away'. She recognized that this was silly but she could not stop herself no matter how hard she tried. 'It's amazing because I used to be so untidy in the past'.

Thought content

Jane said that she was not thin. 'I feel as if I am $8\frac{1}{2}$ stones'. 'When I look in the mirror, I don't look thin'. She liked her abdomen to be 'completely flat' and thought that her 'troublesome' thighs were now 'about right'. She liked seeing her hip bones through her flesh. Jane admitted to hunger at times now, but for most of the past year she said she had not felt hungry at all. She also confided in a dread of seeing a weight increase when she stood on her scales. She said that she ate 'lots' but that she avoided 'unnecessary' foods. These included 'self-indulgent' foods containing sugar and fats. If she ate more than was 'necessary' she felt extremely guilty—'I feel that I am doing something wrong, something that I shouldn't be doing'.

Jane's intake of food was very meagre and identical each day—a 5 oz tin of baked beans, one egg, and crisp breads with cucumber spread. She did not allow her mother to prepare it for her as 'she might try to cheat'. She carefully counted calories and aimed for 'well under 1000 per day'.

Other measures aimed at accelerating her weight loss, apart from exercising excessively, were denied. She had thought about inducing vomiting after eating but decided it was 'too disgusting'. She denied abusing laxatives.

Jane's main preoccupations were with food and weight. 'I guess its on my mind nearly 100 per cent of the time—I think when will I have to eat next, what will I have?'

Abnormal beliefs and interpretation of events

None were elicited apart from ideas related to her weight.

Abnormal experiences

None were elicited.

Cognitive state

She seemed a girl of average intelligence and there were no cognitive deficits on clinical testing.

Patient's appraisal

By the end of the interview, Jane was beginning to admit that she was not completely well. She said that she was easily exhausted and that she had lost interest in her previous activities. She was worried about the fine hair which had grown over her arms and neck. 'I know you think I've got the slimmer's disease—if I do then its not a bad case though—I don't make myself vomit. I used to love food so much. I know I can eat and eat and eat'. Jane was asked what would be the highest weight she could tolerate. 'I don't know. I mightn't mind going up to 7 stones (45 kg)—but definitely no higher'. When she was asked whether she was concerned about her periods stopping she replied, 'I don't mind at all. Its convenient really. It's not like I am trying to have children, is it?' She ended the interview by saying: 'I feel like a hypocrite being here. I don't need anything'.

Physical examination

Jane was very emaciated and weighed 5 st 5 lb (34 kg). Her blood pressure was 100/70 and her pulse was 64. Her periphery was cyanosed. There was lanugo hair over her forearms, the nape of her neck and on the sides of her face.

Interview with informants

Mr and Mrs Morgan were seen together without Jane.

Mrs Morgan confirmed the details of the development of the illness as given by Jane. Both parents commented that Jane had changed dramatically over the past year. She used to be a popular, friendly, good humoured girl who was always 'sensible and obedient' at home. She had always been sensitive about her appearance, particularly her thighs. Father said, however, that she had good reason to worry about her thighs as they were 'on the big side'. Mother disagreed.

Mr Morgan dominated most of the interview. Very distressing for him was Jane's 'lashing out'. 'She has said some very disturbing things to her mother and me even hurtful things. Is it just the food deprivation?' One example of this was when she had said angrily, 'Others have fathers but I don't'. She had never shown feelings like this before. Both parents expressed horror at Jane's weight loss and felt hopeless about their attempts to get her to eat more. They felt they had tried everything.

Mrs Morgan described Rachel's leaving home as 'the last straw'. The sisters had been close at that time and when Rachel left, Jane's weight plummeted.

Both parents remarked on Jane's dependency since she had started losing weight. Mother said that Jane was at her side all day and that she would start crying if she decided to go somewhere alone. Father said that since his return, Jane had clung to him as well—'she lets me hug her now whereas she didn't before'.

Mr Morgan said that he would stay in England as long as necessary to organize Jane's treatment. Mrs Morgan responded to this by saying: 'Yes, but after that you'll go away again'. Mr

Morgan said that he would spend all of his leave entitlement in England until Jane was well again.

As Jane's parents were leaving the room, Mr Morgan dropped back to have a private word with the doctor. He said that one factor in Jane's illness was mother not wanting Jane to leave her. Mother was apparently unhappy being left alone at night. He said that Jane had expressed the desire to gain independence but that she could not because she had to stay and look after mother. The tone of his voice when talking about his ex-wife was obviously critical.

Summary

Jane is a 17-year-old girl who presented with a one year history of severe weight loss. Although the diagnosis of anorexia nervosa and its management by encouraging weight gain appear straightforward in Jane's case, the problem is to gain her co-operation with treatment. In order to do this the psychiatrist requires knowledge of the available treatment options, the likely outcome and, perhaps most important of all, the complex way in which a variety of factors have contributed to Jane's presentation at this time.

Formulation

Diagnosis

The clinical picture is typical of anorexia nervosa. The three criteria which are necessary for the diagnosis are all present.

1. A purposive reduction in food intake (particularly of 'fattening' foods) aimed at reducing weight. Jane's weight has fallen from 54 kg to 34 kg. She has also used other measures to accelerate her weight loss, especially excessive exercise and on one occasion deliberately exacerbated a 'bout of diarrhoea.
2. Amenorrhoea. This is secondary and has been present for six months.
3. A characteristic psychopathology which involves a morbid fear of fatness, a relentless pursuit of thinness and a disturbance of her body image in which she denies abnor-

mality in her size in the face of severe emaciation. Jane gives an unrealistically low weight for the highest she is prepared to countenance reaching.

Jane is in the common age group where anorexia arises and the history is fairly typical. There have been a number of other changes which are frequently seen in conjunction with this disorder. These include a loss of interest in previously enjoyed activities, social withdrawal, depressive feelings, and some obsessional traits. There are no serious differential diagnoses in Jane's case. Organic causes for weight loss are not accompanied by the typical psychopathology evidenced by Jane. Although there were some depressive symptoms these are in part due to her state of self-starvation and they are not sufficient to make a primary diagnosis of a depressive illness. Guilt about eating, loss of interest, early morning waking and eventual exhaustion are very common in anorexia nervosa.

There is also the possibility that Jane has an obsessional disorder. Her premorbid personality had some obsessional features such as her liking for order and routine and these have been accentuated recently. Her need to constantly clear up has the hallmark of an obsessional impulse, in that there was a subjective compulsion which she attempted to resist and which she recognized as being senseless. However, her drive to diet did not have these features. She made no attempt to resist it, nor did she regard it as silly. On the contrary, she valued it highly. It is not unusual for obsessional symptoms to develop in the course of anorexia nervosa and they usually improve with weight restoration. Depressive symptoms behave similarly.

The diagnosis of anorexia nervosa thus appears straightforward.

Aetiology

Anorexia Nervosa usually develops after a period of 'normal' dieting. The more common dieting is in a particular population, the more cases of anorexia nervosa there appear to develop. It is very high, for example, amongst ballet students.

Even before Jane developed her illness, she was sensitive about her appearance. This is suggested by her cosmetic opera-

tion on her forehead and her concern about her thighs. Her
father might have reinforced this by his apparent acceptance that
Jane's thighs were too large and in his pleasure, at least as perceived by Jane, in being surrounded by attractive and healthy
women. These considerations help us to understand why both
Jane and Rachel dieted seriously but not why Jane developed
anorexia nervosa, a condition which has made her both unattrac-
tive and unhealthy. Another factor which might have assisted
Jane in losing a lot of weight initially was her concern with
control. She was conscientious, hard working and self-
controlled, and she probably brought these qualities to bear on
her attempt at weight reduction. It may be that finding other
areas of her life difficult to control, especially interpersonal relationships with her parents and boys (discussed below), she
invested more of her energies in an area which she could control
more readily, her body shape. This could have been facilitated by
a relative insensitivity to internal cues, a secondary effect of
sustained dietary restriction or, as has been suggested by some
authorities, based upon a 'constitutional' predisposing factor to
anorexia nervosa.

There are a variety of possible perpetuating factors for Jane's
illness. Jane's distortion of body image, where she sees herself as
being of normal weight or even fat when she is emaciated,
provides the basis of a vicious cycle. It has been shown that many
patients with anorexia nervosa over-estimate their body size to a
greater extent when they are thin and that their perceptions
become more accurate as they move closer to their healthy
weight.

Other possible effects of the starvation itself need also to be
considered. These include irritability, depression, preoccupation
with food, and impaired concentrations. As a consequence of
these experiences, Jane may feel even less able to cope with her
problems, which may in turn intensify her need to be 'in control'
of her diet.

Jane's history suggests some rivalry between her and her sister.
Since Rachel has not been successful in maintaining a consistent
weight reduction whereas Jane has, she may be loathe to relin-
quish her superiority in this regard.

Although Jane has been popular with her friends and has

managed to do well at her work, she seemed to have some difficulty in coping with her sexual feelings and with boys. She saw sex as 'sinful', feared being fondled, never accepted invitations from boys to go out, and seemed pleased that her periods stopped. Anorexia nervosa may have helped her to cope with this problem by making her look and feel more like a prepubertal girl and less like a sexually mature young woman. Her self-starvation served to flatten her feminine curves, to stop her periods and to extinguish sexual thoughts and feelings. It could be seen as having provided a welcome relief from these issues.

The illness has also ended in Jane's moves to establish independence from her mother. She has become clinging like a small child. Following Rachel's departure from home, Jane's weight fell dramatically. Jane has a very close relationship with her mother and were she to leave home as well then both would be likely to experience a great sense of loss. Mother would then be left alone without anyone to support her. She must have invested much in her children following her separation from Mr Morgan. The pain of such a separation is avoided by Jane's illness. In fact, Jane became again a dependent little girl who needed to be looked after, even fed. In this context, it may be significant that Mrs Morgan has become a child minder at a time when her daughters are likely to leave home. This may be the role in which she feels most comfortable. Rachel's departure to join Mr Morgan may have generated fears in Mrs Morgan that Jane will do the same and this would add to her sense of loss. Father's comment to the doctor that Mrs Morgan fears being left alone might have a strong element of truth.

Mr Morgan has maintained a close contact with his family despite 15 years of separation. From both Mrs Morgan's comments to her husband during their interview with the doctor as well as Jane's account, it seems likely that she would like her ex-husband back again. Jane's illness heightened his involvement with the family and in part it may be perpetuated by its serving to reconstitute the family around the crisis it engendered.

The discussion above suggests that a variety of influences may be at work in shaping Jane's illness. These include factors understandable at physiological, psychological, interpersonal and socio-cultural levels.

Further investigations

Further investigations aimed at evaluating Jane's physical status should be undertaken. It is important to assess her serum electrolytes since a hypokalaemic alkalosis would suggest that she is secretly inducing vomiting. A number of abnormalities might be revealed in a full blood examination, liver function tests, etc. but these are of uncertain significance in anorexia nervosa and are likely to be the result of the self-starvation. Luteinizing hormone (LH), follicle-stimulating hormone (FSH), and oestrogen assays will be low but they are not essential investigations.

More important, from the point of view of management, will be a fuller assessment of the psychological and family factors discussed under aetiology. The importance of the observations already made can be further supported or perhaps rejected following more interviews with Jane and with her family.

Management

In all patients with anorexia nervosa the essential short-term goal is weight restoration with the longer-term goal of maintenance of a healthy weight. Experience shows that psychotherapeutic measures are generally not effective until the patient is restored to a reasonable weight. The consequences which the patient fears, and which need to be tackled in treatment are avoided and less clearly manifest when she is emaciated.

Left to her own devices, Jane would not be expected to gain a substantial amount of weight. It might be possible for her mother, with a great deal of support from the doctor, to put pressure on Jane to eat more. However, the simplest and most certain means of ensuring weight gain is by admission to hospital where Jane can be supervised and supported by nursing and medical staff. The initial obstacle to treating Jane will be to get her to accept admission.

Although she has not accepted that she is emaciated and that she needs help, her statements during the interview suggested some uncertainty about this. She admitted to a number of distressing feelings and these can be built on by the doctor to gain her co-operation. In addition, he will probably have the co-operation of her parents in putting pressure on her to accept admission. He will need to be firm and insistent that this is the proper course to take. At the same time he will need to make it clear to Jane that although he understands her fears of weight gain this will be essential if she is to be helped with some of the underlying problems that trouble her. Some more interviews may be necessary to persuade Jane to accept admission. If this should prove impossible then resort to admission under compulsory order will need to be considered as Jane's condition is a life-threatening one. In practice this rarely proves necessary.

The in-patient phase of treatment will be directed to restoring Jane to a healthy weight, somewhere in the region of her pre-morbid weight of 54 kg. It will require skilled nursing care to achieve this and to overcome her resistance to weight gain. Success will be most likely with nurses who understand the condition well. She will need a nurse to supervise her meals and be with her for most of the day. The nurses must be able to demonstrate a combination of firmness and sympathy. Previous experience with such cases is invaluable.

Jane needs to gain about 20 kg and this will require about two months in hospital. When she nears her healthy weight she will be given increasing opportunities to eat unsupervised and she will eventually have weekends at home. A strict 'behavioural' regime is not necessary, nor, given experienced nursing, is tube feeding.

During the course of her stay in hospital further meetings with her and her family will be aimed at gaining a better understanding of her difficulties and in the light of this to plan management following her discharge. She will probably need follow-up treatment as an out-patient for at least a year. The potential benefits of individual psychotherapy or family therapy will need to be assessed. The follow-up treatment will be directed at helping Jane to maintain her weight and to help her resolve those problems which have been previously 'solved' by self-starvation.

Prognosis

In the short term the prognosis for weight gain is good. It is likely that Jane will eventually accept admission to hospital and in hospital she will be restored to a near healthy weight. It is also likely that Jane's attitude to her body and her depressive feelings will improve. The effects of the malnutrition itself on Jane's physical and mental state is important and, when reversed, is likely to result in a major improvement. Although she is likely to restart menstruation after she achieves her expected weight, this may be delayed for a number of months.

The long-term prognosis is more difficult to assess. A number of factors in Jane's case would suggest a good prognosis. The history is relatively short, being about one year. A 'long' history in this condition would be regarded as one of three years or more. Anorexia nervosa arising in a girl of Jane's age usually has a better prognosis than in an older girl. Another good prognostic point is Jane's good premorbid social adjustment in terms of interpersonal relationships and work. This usually has an important bearing on the eventual outcome. Finally, the absence of bulimic episodes and self-induced vomiting also suggest a good outcome.

Overall, the known prognostic features for this condition all point to an eventual recovery in Jane's case.

Brief formulation

Jane is a 17-year-old girl who presents with a one-year history of severe weight loss.

Diagnosis

The clinical picture is typical of anorexia nervosa. There is a deliberate restriction of diet, the characteristic psychopathology (a pursuit of thinness, a morbid fear of putting on weight, and a denial of emaciation) and secondary amenorrhoea. Other features of Jane's mental state, particularly depression and obsessionality, are also frequently seen in this disorder.

Aetiology

Jane's illness followed a period of 'normal dieting' in response to fairly common adolescent concerns. Contributing to the progression from normal dieting to morbid food restriction were probably Jane's determination, capacity for self-control, and possibly an abnormal ability to 'deny' or be insensitive to hunger. There are a number of likely perpetuating factors including a vicious circle in which the thinner she becomes, the more she overestimates her size. Jane may welcome a relief from sexual feelings that starvation brings and her illness may also serve as an important family function in halting her moves to independence, thus keeping her as a 'little girl' for her mother who may fear being left alone.

Further investigations

Jane's physical status should be carefully assessed but a search for 'physical causes' of weight loss will prove unrewarding. Further interviews with Jane and with her family will help to clarify some of the likely aetiological factors described above.

Management

The priority is for Jane to gain weight. Attempts at psychotherapy before this is achieved are unlikely to be successful. Reversal of the malnutrition in addition to saving life, will also ameliorate the effects of starvation on Jane's mental state.

Weight gain in Jane's case will require admission to hospital and the doctor and parents will need to persuade her to accept this. This is likely to be achieved after a few out-patient sessions. In hospital good nursing care and firm but sympathetic handling should result in a steady weight gain and restoration to a near normal weight over a period of two months or so. At the same time the foundations for a psychotherapeutic relationship should be laid. Jane will probably require continued treatment for some time after discharge from hospital to help her with the problems which have contributed to her illness. The family will probably need to be involved in this treatment.

Prognosis

Admission should result in weight gain and a considerable improvement in Jane's mental state. For the long term the prognosis appears favourable on account of the short history of the illness, the young age of onset, and Jane's good premorbid adjustment.

Further information

Jane accepted admission to hospital after the first interview, to give her 'parents a rest'. She was in fact admitted to a unit which specializes in the treatment of anorexia nervosa and there were no particular difficulties in ensuring that Jane reached 54 kg. She was in hospital for 10 weeks altogether but lost some weight during two weekends at home. Her weight on discharge was 51 kg. All physical investigations were normal apart from the expected low LH, FSH and oestrogen levels. At the time of her discharge Jane said that she felt a lot 'healthier' and more cheerful. She admitted, however, that she felt 'fat' at 51 kg and that she would like to lose 'about half a stone' (3 kg).

During her stay in hospital Jane was seen regularly on an individual basis. Her displeasure with her weight gain was very evident as was her reluctance to talk about other aspects of her life. Sullen nods were a frequent response to questions put to her. Mr Morgan returned to the United States two weeks after Jane's admission to hospital and he was due to come back to England for two weeks three months later. Sessions with Jane's mother supported the view that there was a marked interdependence between them and that this was an important contributing factor to Jane's illness. Their relationship seemed to require Jane to be a 'little girl'.

In view of the prominent family factors and of Jane's reluctance to engage in individual therapy, it was decided that following discharge Jane would be seen together with her mother, with her father and Rachel attending when they were in England.

In the first three months of follow-up treatment a number of important hypotheses were explored which presented Jane's symptoms as serving a function in maintaining the current family system. It was evident that Jane's symptoms prevented her from leaving home and her mother, whom she saw as needing to be looked after. Mother had a fear that Jane would follow Rachel and go and live with father. It was learnt that before Rachel left her mother she had behaved in a seriously delinquent manner so that her move to her father was virtually forced on mother because of her inability to control the girl. Jane's symptoms also served to keep father involved with his family in mutual concern with his ex-wife. It appeared at times that Jane wished that the family could be reconstituted so that she could leave home without her mother being left entirely on her own. In the four sessions, when Mr Morgan or Rachel were also present, it was very obvious that both undermined Mrs Morgan's confidence and authority with Jane. Mrs Morgan was made to look incompetent.

During this period Jane lost weight rapidly and dropped to 35 kg. The psychiatrist's attempts to put mother in charge of Jane failed, as did interventions aimed at increasing Jane's independence from her mother. It seemed likely that Jane would need readmission soon.

Jane's anorexia has been managed within the context of her family and information emerging through the use of this approach has led to some alterations of the original aetiological hypotheses. However, she has deteriorated in spite of the psychiatrist's interventions. The reader is invited to reformulate Jane's problem in order to develop a more useful management strategy.

Reformulation

Diagnosis

This remains anorexia nervosa.

Aetiology

It is necessary to establish what factors have perpetuated Jane's symptoms. It seems likely that family factors have been important in this, and an attempt has been made to tackle these. The main focus has been on Jane's and mother's interdependence. Mother appears to fear the loss of Jane and Jane fears the consequences of leaving her mother. The manner of Rachel's leaving home is noteworthy; she had become unmanageable by her mother and had to be transferred to her father's care. It is likely that father wishes to have both his daughters living with him, and his undermining of his ex-wife's authority over Jane makes her appear incompetent to care for her, as was the case with Rachel before. This might require Jane's going to live with father. Jane's illness ties her in dependence on her mother but also could provide a justification for father taking her away to be better looked after. Jane thus appears to be caught up in a tussle between her parents.

However, interventions directed to the mutual dependence of Jane and mother have not had any impact on Jane's condition. It could be that they were not very skilfully executed but it also might be helpful to rethink the situation and change the focus.

An important effect of Jane's illness has been to keep father in contact with mother, to 'reconstitute' the family of old. Although this might be seen as an understandable hope in the child of a divorced couple, it is unusual for such a wish to be maintained for 15 years, unless one or both of the parents have failed to accept the meaning of their divorce. There is some evidence that Mrs Morgan is the one who may have failed to come to terms with this. Jane has said that she felt her mother still missed her father and it may be remembered that Mrs Morgan expressed resentment about her ex-husband's impending return to the United States. In contrast, the significant loss incurred in the divorce for Mr Morgan has not been his wife but his children. His continued contact with the family has been based on them.

Management

It follows from this line of thinking that the relationship between mother and father should receive more consideration particularly mother's inability to divorce 'emotionally' her husband. Her feelings of loss need to be addressed and a relationship between the couple established which does not involve Jane as a fulcrum. Mrs Morgan will also need support and encouragement to withstand her ex-husband's undermining manoeuvres and this may help her in dealing with her fears that Jane will leave her for him.

If Jane continues to lose weight in spite of these interventions then she will need to be re-admitted to hospital and a new management strategy developed.

Further investigations

Jane's weight will continue to need monitoring.

The psychiatrist will need to observe closely the effect of his interventions on Jane and on her family. Their responses will determine whether he pursues the management outlined above, whether and how he modifies it or whether he abandons it.

Prognosis

If this formulation is correct than Jane should begin to improve. However, because of the hypothesized family dynamics, any improvement in Jane is likely to be met by a resistance within the family. In his case it might be expected that her father would make stronger efforts to undermine his ex-wife.

Postscript

The psychiatrist undertook the management outlined above and spent a considerable period of time exploring and underlining Mrs Morgan's strengths. The loss of her husband was discussed at some length and means were explored for her to negotiate a direct relationship with him which did not involve Jane. As a result of this she began to exercise more control over Jane's eating. However, as Jane began to gain weight Mr Morgan made an open attempt to get her away from his ex-wife. He said that the treatment was ineffective and he had therefore made arrangements for Jane to be seen by a specialist in Los Angeles whose treatment would be more effective. Mrs Morgan had by now sufficient authority to resist her ex-husband's plans and Jane decided that she could not live with a father who was 'so domineering'.

Over the next four months Jane continued to gain weight and nine months after discharge she had reached 45 kg. She found a new job which she enjoyed and began to go out with a boyfriend. Jane was now able to discuss her uncertainties about the latter with her mother and in therapy sessions. A friend also offered to share a flat with her but Jane was uncertain about this. Although her mother said it was 'probably a good idea', her tone of voice showed that she was clearly unhappy about the possibility. Eventually Jane left to decide for herself and she opted to stay at home for the 'time being'.

Treatment was ended as Jane maintained a steady weight of 50 kg and it was believed that she and her mother could resolve any remaining issues. She had still not begun to menstruate.

5

A drinking problem—the case of Mr Pillay, aged 46

Presenting complaint

Mr Pillay was a 46-year-old Mauritian of Indian extraction who was referred to the Department of psychological medicine in a general hospital following his admission to a general ward. He had been admitted from the accident and emergency department following a 'blackout' in a photographic laboratory where he worked. He was found deeply unconscious by a workmate but had sustained no injury.

The following account of the admission was given by the referring physician.

On arrival at the hospital Mr Pillay was found to be pyrexial, shivering, agitated, tremulous, and disorientated and was diagnosed as suffering from a chest infection and an acute confusional state. On admission to the ward he showed clouding of consciousness, difficulty in attending to questions and an inability to register what was going on about him. He was grossly disorientated for time and place. Physical examination revealed a temperature of 39°C and evidence of consolidation of the lungs. A chest X-ray revealed a picture of bronchopneumonia.

Mr Pillay remained confused for the next three days. He was found to wander around the ward looking for 'the singers' and complained that people were 'getting' at him. One nurse was accused of administering poisons to him. Treatment with ampicillin for the chest infection was accompanied by a resolution of the fever and in addition he was sedated with chlormethiazole for five days.

On the fourth day he was able to give a history. At this stage he admitted to drinking 'two pints of beer and one eighth of a bottle of whisky' per day. Liver function tests showed a raised γ-GT level (45 i.u./l). (Normal range at the laboratory would be 4–35 i.u./l.) Mr Pillay was seen on the medical ward by a social worker. He complained to her of problems at work but said that otherwise he had no difficulties in his life. He said that he had many friends, 'too many', and that drinking would not be a problem in the future. An appointment was offered for the psychiatric out-patient department two weeks later and Mr Pillay accepted it to reassure everyone that everything was all right. He was subsequently discharged from his in-patient stay.

Mr Pillay arrived for his out-patient appointment and the following history was obtained.

Mr Pillay had few complaints. Those that he had were exclusively concerned with his work as a technician in a dark-room. The air conditioner had recently broken down and after sharing a confined space with two co-workers for a day he felt 'jittery' and also felt that his head was 'exploding'.

A more detailed drinking history was obtained. Mr Pillay said that he had been drinking regularly from the age of 19 but that his intake had increased over the past six years since he had started his current job. The amount of alcohol which he admitted consuming was as stated during his stay on the ward. On occasions, though, he said he might have drunk a quarter of a bottle of spirits. Mr Pillay admitted to a morning drink 'rarely' and also to some morning tremulousness and dry retching 'occasionally', although more frequently over the past few months. He denied any 'black-outs' in the past or any lapses of memory. Mr Pillay said he normally drank every day but when he developed a cough and fever with his chest infection he stopped. This was a few days before his admission to hospital. Since discharge from the hospital 10 days earlier he said he had drunk three beers but no spirits.

Family history

Mr Pillay's father was aged 76 and a plantation manager in Mauritius. Although fit, Mr Pillay described him as a 'very heavy drinker'. His mother was aged 68 and well.

Mr Pillay had two brothers and one sister. Both his brothers were in Mauritius and one was older than the patient. They were both successful in their careers, one a civil servant and the other an accountant. His sister, aged 34, was the youngest child and she lived with her husband and two children in London, a few miles from the patient's home.

Mr Pillay said his family was a close one and that relationships had always been harmonious. He spoke of his parents in idealistic terms. He said he was brought up with much 'love, care, and affection'. Correspondence was regular but Mr Pillay had not visited Mauritius since his arrival in England six years previously. He said that he saw his sister most weekends until three months previously when she had had her second child.

There was no family history of mental disorder and his father had never required medical attention because of his drinking. An uncle mentioned, now dead from a cause unknown to the patient, was also a heavy drinker.

Personal history

There had been some complications surrounding Mr Pillay's birth. He did not know their exact nature but he remembered being told that little hope had been held for his survival.

Apart from this, his childhood had been unremarkable. He had a tendency to keep to himself. He said his family had regarded him as 'independent' from an early age and had commented on a 'stubborn streak' in his make-up.

Mr Pillay went to a highly regarded private school in Mauritius and matriculated at the age of 19. He was a serious and ambitious student who was expected to do well in the future.

On leaving school Mr Pillay went to work in the civil service. After five years he became private secretary to a government minister, a post which he held for four years. He then moved to a merchant bank where he held an administrative position of some responsibility for 10 years. Then, at the age of 39, Mr Pillay left the bank, for reasons which he explained vaguely, one of them being a change of location.

At this time Mr Pillay decided to come to England where his sister was already living. For the first year after his arrival he worked as an interior decorator but with only modest success. He said that he had always had a special interest in, and flair for, design. Mr Pillay obtained his present job as a laboratory technician in a specialist photographic firm six years previously through the agency of a friend. This laboratory dealt with high quality photographic reproduction and Mr Pillay worked mainly in a highly organized darkroom. For the past year or so he had apparently become less enthusiastic about his work and often complained about the cramped and stuffy conditions. He had suggested a number of possible improvements but to no avail. Mr Pillay said that his employers were very satisfied with his work and that his job had never been threatened. Mr Pillay had never married because the idea of marriage had never appealed to him. He had, however, had a number of short-lived affairs which he termed 'illicit' as some had been with married women. He did not have a current lady friend.

He lived in a rented flat which he had decorated himself and of which he was proud. He said that he was a 'gregarious' man who had 'lots of friends'. The impression was given that they drank together although he was at pains to point out that none were excessive drinkers.

Past medical history

Mr Pillay said that he had had malaria when he was seven years old and viral pneumonia when aged 26. He also had an episode of 'rheumatic pains' in the legs a year previously for which he did not seek treatment.

Past psychiatric history

None was elicited.

Previous personality

Mr Pillay described himself as a 'slightly nervous' man who generally felt in control of his life. He denied ever feeling low spirited. He said that he tended to become 'impatient if things are not done right'. This somewhat perfectionistic trait had led him to complain about the organization of the laboratory at work. Mr Pillay spent much time in meticulously decorating his flat. He described decoration and carpentry as his main interests and he was frequently employed by acquaintances to do odd jobs of this kind. He indicated that he expected a high standard of moral behaviour from other people and that he tried to maintain similar high standards for himself. Mr Pillay said that he found it difficult to assert himself and tended to back down in arguments. He used to read novels but had not done so for about a year or so. Although brought up as a Christian he was a non-believer as he could find no 'convincing evidence' to support such a belief.

Mr Pillay had never been in trouble with the police. He smoked 30–40 cigarettes per day and he denied taking any illicit drugs.

Physical examination

This was not performed. On discharge from hospital no abnormal signs were found.

Mental state

Appearance and general behaviour

Mr Pillay was a small, good-looking, thin man with his hair immaculately combed in such a way as to conceal an advanced state of baldness. He was well spoken and pleasant at all times and displayed an unusually deferential manner to the psychiatrist, frequently addressing him as 'sir'.

During the interview he was politely evasive and gave the impression that he was painting a brighter picture than the real one. Most questions touching on potentially sensitive areas (such as leaving Mauritius or sexual feelings) were answered briefly or side-tracked into less emotionally charged ones. This was done in an ostensibly respectful manner but his obvious discomfort and reluctance made it clear to the interviewer that further probing at this stage would not prove rewarding. There was a powerful sense that only issues lying close to the surface were to be discussed.

Mr Pillay was observed to be almost constantly fidgety and uncomfortable.

Talk

This was fluent and spontaneous.

Mood

Mr Pillay denied any depressive feelings and said he was optimistic about the future. He expressed no feelings of self reproach. He admitted to feeling tense at times but made light of this. Somatic accompaniments to his anxiety were denied.

Thought content

This was mainly concerned with difficulties at work which he believed could now be remedied. The employer, he said, was finally taking some notice of his complaints.

Abnormal beliefs and interpretation of events

There were none currently but Mr Pillay vaguely recalled harbouring the belief that he was the subject of persecution during his hospital admission.

Cognitive state

Cognitive testing revealed no abnormality of memory or intellectual functioning. Digit span up to seven numbers forwards and five numbers backwards was executed without difficulty. A name and address were perfectly recalled after five minutes and Mr Pillay was very well informed about current news events.

Appraisal of illness

When the subject of alcohol was raised Mr Pillay conceded that he might have been drinking too much but he was now confident that it would never be a problem again. He believed that the symptoms necessitating his admission to hospital were entirely the result of his chest infection and claimed that no one had ever told him that they might be related to alcohol. The suggestion that these were the symptoms of alcohol addiction and withdrawal seemed to surprise him. Armed with this new knowledge, he said, he would be even more determined to control his drinking.

When it was suggested that he might have a drinking problem and that abstinence was the wisest course on which to embark, Mr Pillay said that he could not accept the idea of stopping alcohol completely. At times he gave indications that he was unsure about whether he needed help. The idea was never totally dismissed but when he was asked to specify what he might need help with, he talked mainly about problems in the dark-room. When asked whether he was content with the way he was managing other aspects of his life he answered affirmatively.

At the end of the interview Mr Pillay was asked whether he minded if the doctor spoke to his sister in order to learn more about his situation. He replied that he did not wish to 'burden' her with his problem, especially as she had recently had a baby. After further discussion he obstinately but politely forbad any contact. He also said that he did not want to impose on his friends and that he would be unhappy if his employer were to know any details of his troubles.

Summary

Mr Pillay is a 46-year-old man referred following admission to a medical ward because of a 'black-out' and the development of a seriously disturbed mental state. His symptoms resolved after a few days and he was referred to a psychiatrist for an assessment of his drinking behaviour.

Having clarified the importance of alcohol in his presentation the fundamental difficulty confronting the psychiatrist is to communicate his understanding of the problems of alcohol dependence to Mr Pillay in such a way as to facilitate his maximum co-operation with treatment.

Formulation

Diagnosis

The clinical picture displayed by Mr Pillay on admission to the ward was typical of an acute organic confusional state. For two to three days his consciousness was clouded, he was disorientated in time and place, he was unable to register events going on about him and there was also evidence of agitation, auditory hallucinations and fleeting persecutory delusions. In Mr Pillay's case there was an obvious physical disorder, namely bronchopneumonia. However, this is unlikely to cause such a florid confusional state as this, except in the very young and the aged.

It is likely in Mr Pillay's case that alcohol was playing an

important role. Withdrawal from alcohol in a physically dependent person may result in an acute confusional state termed
delirium tremens. Mr Pillay's drinking has certainly been sustained for many years and this is supported by the raised α-GT
level in his liver function tests. He admitted to morning tremulousness 'occasionally' and this is an early feature of physical
dependence on alcohol. Dry retching in the morning also points
to excessive alcohol consumption. The 'black-out' was not
witnessed but it is likely that this was an epileptic fit. He was
found to be deeply unconscious and was afterwards confused.
Convulsions often usher in the florid mental disturbances of
delirium tremens. The history suggests also that Mr Pillay, as a
consequence of his chest infection, had reduced his alcohol
intake so that he was experiencing a state of relative withdrawal
from alcohol. The marked agitation and tremulousness observed
are part of the picture of delirium tremens.

Mr Pillay is either underestimating his consumption of alcohol
or he is dissimulating. His failure to recall the fact that he had
been told that his symptoms were associated with alcohol points
to an ability on his part to 'deny' unpleasant memories. The
personal history he gave was a superficial one and this makes the
search for other evidence of a drinking problem, such as a
history of psychological or social impairment, difficult. There are
a few clues but their interpretation involves a large degree of
inference. In general terms there is the appearance of a decline in
Mr Pillay's life. This is perhaps most evident in his work history.
After doing well at school he seemed to occupy responsible jobs
in government and later, in a bank, which called for the exercise
of administrative skills. He then left Mauritius for reasons which
are obscure and he now finds himself in the relatively unskilled
position of a dark-room technician. One recalls here that he was
an ambitious and hard working young man and one also wonders
whether his departure from Mauritius was related to a drinking
problem even then. This suspicion is strengthened by Mr Pillay's
vague account of why he left. It is difficult to gauge from the
history whether there has been a deterioration in his personal
relationships. The 'rheumatic pains' that he described as having
occurred a year ago were possibly the calf tenderness which
alcoholics commonly experience.

There is no evidence that Mr Pillay suffers from a psychiatric illness, such as depression, to which his drinking might be secondary.

To summarize, Mr Pillay has suffered from an episode of acute organic confusion in which alcohol withdrawal has played a major role with a contribution from a chest infection. There is evidence that he drinks excessively and that he is physically dependent on alcohol. There is lesser evidence of a social decline which might have been a consequence of drinking. Apart from some evidence of liver damage on admission to hospital there were no other physical or neuropsychiatric complications.

Aetiology

Those factors causing the acute confusional state have already been discussed above. The precise pathophysiology caused by excessive drinking and which results in delirium tremens is unknown. Most cases commence two to three days after abstinence from alcohol and may be preceded by one or a series of epileptic fits. There is a significant association between delirium tremens and physical disorders, pneumonia, as in Mr Pillay's case, being a common example. One may predispose to the development of the other. Alcoholic tremulousness is also a symptom of alcohol withdrawal which occurs after a short period of abstinence, even overnight. Morning nausea and vomiting are usually attributed to alcoholic gastritis but it is possible that they may also be of central nervous system origin and related to withdrawal.

The fact that Mr Pillay has shown evidence of a physical dependence on alcohol indicates that he drinks heavily and that this has been sustained for a long time. The history obtained is not a very satisfactory one in terms of the information it provides which might have a bearing on aetiological factors. Few facts have been adduced which are helpful in understanding why Mr Pillay drinks heavily and one is forced at this stage to make a number of inferences which receive only limited support.

There is a family history of heavy drinking in Mr Pillay's father and uncle. There is some evidence of a genetic predisposition to the development of physical dependence on alcohol, but this is difficult to disentangle from the psychological influences existing in a home where a parent is a heavy drinker. A familial transmission of heavy drinking is, however, common.

Mr Pillay does not appear to have been drinking heavily as a consequence of a psychiatric disorder such as depression. One looks, therefore, for personality vulnerabilities or difficult life circumstances which might predispose him to seek gratification, or relief of tension in alcohol. With someone who has a long drinking history it is often difficult to distinguish difficulties which lead to drinking as opposed to those which are a consequence of drinking. Comment has already been made on Mr Pillay's work record. It is possible that the decline noted was a consequence of excessive drinking but it is also possible that a failure to achieve the success he wished for, due perhaps to personal limitations, might have led him to drink more.

Mr Pillay described some personality traits which could be seen as potentially causing difficulties. He said that he tended to be an anxious man and his tension was indeed obvious during the interview. The frustration he felt if things were not 'right' seems to be related to some perfectionist traits in his personality. This may well have contributed to some of his difficulties at work where a mixture of impatience and unassertiveness appear to have inhibited him from acting more forcefully on his complaints. His inappropriately deferential manner which was such a striking feature during the interview was consistent with his view of himself as someone who had difficulties in self-assertion.

Mr Pillay's social situation is problematical. He claimed to have many friends, yet he gave the impression of being an isolated man. It is difficult to specify where this impression derives from but a number of factors suggesting this have emerged. He described himself as a 'loner' in childhood. A specific friend was never mentioned during the interview, nor was there ever any reference to the other people having any impact on his life. He gave the impression of being a very private person. This is consistent with his finding marriage undesirable and the absence of any long-term heterosexual relationships. The main supportive figure in his life seemed to have been his sister with whom he spent most weekends. The fact that she had a baby recently might have a bearing on his having presented at this time since it is conceivable that she might have withdrawn some support from him as a result of this. It is noteworthy that she never made contact with a doctor to discuss her brother's condition. Perhaps she did not even known about his illness. Finally, Mr Pillay appeared during the interview to be someone who could not relate comfortably to the doctor. Although allowance needs to be made for the threatening nature of an interview with a psychiatrist, Mr Pillay's difficulties seemed to be more profound. His defensiveness, although polite, made it difficult to warm to him. He gave the impression of detached aloofness and of inexperience in talking about himself with others. There was a striking absence of an easy social competence.

Many of the factors discussed above which may have a bearing on Mr Pillay's drinking are speculative in view of the meagre information available. However, it is helpful to think about these as some of the ideas raised will guide the psychiatrist in the type of information he will seek when the next opportunity presents itself.

Further investigations

There is clearly a need for more personal details. The exact extent to which alcohol has salience in his life is unclear. Also the course of his life history and the effect that drinking has had on his work and social relationships need further exploration. Evidence is also necessary to evaluate the postulated role of personality factors in predisposing him to drink excessively. An informant, particularly his sister, would be the most helpful source of information but at present she is barred by the patient from helping. One will have to rely therefore on what can be learnt from further interviews with the patient himself.

A repeat of the liver function tests should be performed to check whether the γ-GT level has returned to normal.

More detailed psychological testing for cognitive impairment should be considered as might a CT scan. This would provide measures against which future testing might reveal deterioration. Any impairment demonstrated should be discussed with Mr Pillay since it might increase his motivation for treatment.

Management

The major difficulty is Mr Pillay's apparent lack of motivation to seek help. The details of any treatment can only be worked out if he makes a commitment to give up drinking and this aim would be much more realistic if he could establish a therapeutic alliance with the doctor.

The absence of information about the extent to which drinking has interfered with Mr Pillay's life makes it difficult to decide on how much pressure should be exerted on him to accept treatment. He denies a significant impact on his level of functioning, although there is good evidence that he is physically dependent on alcohol. Because of this, one would want to encourage him to make a more realistic appraisal of his difficulties. Mr Pillay's failure to disclose important details is an important limitation in this task. There is a temptation to challenge him by saying that he is not very concerned to co-operate, to discharge him, and to suggest that he will be back soon enough.

However, another attempt might be made to enlist his co-operation. For this to have any hope of success, special attention will need to be paid to the relationship made with him and this will need to take account of some of the observations already discussed. The interviewer will have to be on his guard against reacting to the patient's contradictory submissive stubborness with impatience. He will need to respect Mr Pillay's privacy. The best approach might involve an implicit indication that the interview is not 'psychological' but 'factual'. Fewer 'why did that happen?' questions and more 'what happened then?' questions might help to create a 'fact finding' atmosphere. The aim would be to construct a picture of an average day in Mr Pillay's life: what he does and with whom, when he drinks and what. 'Feelings' should be left out. At the end of the session a joint appraisal could be made of the 'facts of the case' and the patient invited to draw logical conclusions. Mr Pillay spoke a number of times during his first interview about 'facts' so that this approach might speak to him in a language which is congruent with his way of viewing the world. It is also important to inform him of the complications, physical, psychological and social which he risks with continued drinking.

If Mr Pillay were to agree to treatment it is difficult at this stage to suggest which type of treatment would prove most helpful to him. The treatment needs to be tailored to his particular needs and these are not clear. The goal should be abstinence in view of this physical dependence on alcohol. Long-term supportive measures will be necessary to help him achieve this and their nature would also depend on a fuller assessment of his specific difficulties. For example, he might need some help towards greater assertiveness in dealing with others which might reduce his feelings of frustration. Antabuse or Alcoholics Anonymous might also play a role although given his social unease, the latter might not prove acceptable to him.

If Mr Pillay elects not to accept the offer of treatment then it would be reasonable to leave him with the invitation to refer himself back if he should change his mind in the future.

Prognosis

A confident prognosis cannot be given. However, unless Mr Pillay can change his attitude to his drinking it is likely that it will continue and that further complications such as withdrawal symptoms and liver damage will occur. Quite apart from his own lack of incentive to abstain is the apparent absence of people in his life who might encourage him to stop drinking. Although Mr Pillay has apparently shown some ability to control his drinking in the past, as he has been able to maintain his job without interruption, it is very likely, if he continues in the same vein, that more problems will arise.

This admission to hospital, however, may represent the first occasion on which Mr Pillay has had to confront his drinking. There is a small chance that it may result in a significant change in his behaviour without anyone else's help.

Brief formulation

Mr Pillay is a 46-year-old man referred to a psychiatrist following admission to hospital following a 'black-out' and the development of a bizarre mental state.

Diagnosis

Mr Pillay has had an acute organic brain syndrome (confusional state). His mental state on admission was typical of this condition, with clouding of consciousness, disorientation, agitation, hallucinations and delusional ideas. Two factors contributed to this episode—a chest infection and alcohol withdrawal. There is good evidence that Mr Pillay drinks excessively and that he is physically dependent on alcohol.

Aetiology

The organic basis of the acute confusion has already been mentioned. There is no clear-cut psychiatric illness to which alcohol dependence is secondary. A family history of heavy drinking may indicate a genetic predisposition or some type of 'psychological transmission'. The superficial history obtained from the patient makes the assessment of personality vulnerabilities difficult but there is some evidence of excessive tension, perfectionistic traits and absence of self-assertiveness. An impression was gained of social isolation.

Further investigation

More personal details are required but Mr Pillay was reluctant to offer these and has barred access to an informant. Liver function tests need to be repeated and consideration given to more extensive testing of cognitive functions.

Management

The major problem at this stage is to engage Mr Pillay's co-operation with treatment. To establish a satisfactory treatment alliance will require special attention to the relationship made with him. If he agrees to co-operate more whole-heartedly then more definitive treatment plans can be made which will be tailored to his particular needs. The goal will be abstinence and its achievement will require long-term supportive measures and attention to specific personal difficulties. If he elects not to accept treatment he should be offered the opportunity to refer himself back in the future.

Prognosis

It is likely that he will continue to drink and that further complications will arise. Further episodes of delerium tremens and more severe liver damage are to be expected, as are new physical and neuropsychiatric complications. This admission to hospital may however, represent the first occasion on which Mr Pillay has had to confront his drinking problem and there is a small chance that it may result in a significant change in his behaviour without anyone else's help.

Further information

Mr Pillay was given an appointment to return to the clinic one month later. The Christmas period intervened between the first and second visits.

When he was next seen in the clinic he said that he was very well except that he was 'virtually compelled' by his friends to have a 'brandy or two' over Christmas. He admitted also to a pint of Guinness on another occasion but was adamant that he had consumed no more. He remarked that he felt much better, that his appetite had improved, and that he was now eating breakfast after getting up with a 'clear mind'. He said that his work situation had improved and a new rota had been established. His colleagues had been supportive and urged him to go out for a walk when 'the cell' became too stuffy.

Mr Pillay had avoided his firm's Christmas parties and said that if he 'put his mind to it' he could live without alcohol. In the evenings he had visited his sister or his friends. They knew about his problems now and they avoided drinking in his presence.

Mr Pillay said that he did not need any further help but agreed to come again in three months time to make sure that everything was all right. The pathology report indicated that his liver function tests had reverted to normal.

Three months later he was seen again. He said that he felt well and had no problems. He admitted to a drink 'about every week'. On one occasion a relative visited from Moscow with some 'special vodka' and he felt he 'had to drink a few glasses'. He was strongly advised to abstain completely but he said this was not necessary as he was fully in control. Mr Pillay was discharged from the clinic but was told that he could refer himself back if any problems arose.

During both interviews Mr Pillay's mental state was similar to that of the first interview apart from a more marked insistence on his part that there was no longer a problem. By insisting there was no problem he made it difficult to explore further any facet of his life, whatever the emphasis chosen. The frame of reference of the interviews was shifted to that of a confirmation that all was well, rather than an exploration of what could be done to help. Any suggestion that there might be a problem or questions which might have hinted that a problem was suspected were made to appear somehow impertinent. The psychiatrist decided to respect Mr Pillay's integrity and hoped that a sufficiently good engagement was made to enable him to return for help if this should prove necessary.

Four months later, Mr Pillay referred himself back to the clinic. He said 'I had a few drinks and then went berserk'. He felt ill and described visual hallucinations of 'hideous animals'. A marked tremor was evident and he was very apprehensive. Mr Pillay however was not confused and he was normally orientated in time and place. He was admitted to a psychiatric hospital with a diagnosis of 'acute alcoholic hallucinosis'.

Mr Pillay was an in-patient for four weeks. A physical examination performed on admission showed an enlarged tender liver and a definite impairment of sensation below the ankles, but normal ankles jerks. Investigations revealed abnormal liver function tests (γ-GT 66 i.u./l; AST 44 i.u./l) (the normal range in the laboratory would be 7 to 40 i.u./l). Alcohol withdrawal was covered with a chlormethiazole regime and in addition he was given multivitamin supplements. On the ward he was observed to be a quiet, shy man who never initiated conversations with others. Very little further information about his past history was elicited although he later admitted to drinking a half bottle of vodka per day for a few weeks before admission. He was noted to have no visitors. After two weeks in hospital he slipped out on a number of occasions and admitted to having had a 'few drinks'.

He was discharged from hospital much improved in his physical and mental state and was to be followed up in the out-patient department. However, he attended only once. On that occasion he claimed he was well and no longer drinking. His attitude was very similar to the one he had shown when he was first seen. On physical examination he had no signs of a peripheral neuropathy. Mr Pillay did not keep his next appointment.

Five months later, Mr Pillay was brought by a work colleague to the accident and emergency department of the hospital. He smelt of alcohol, was tremulous, ataxic, and disorientated and appeared to be hallucinating. He was again admitted to hospital and again withdrawn from alcohol. A diagnosis of delirium tremens was made. A week after admission he developed an episode of acute pancreatitis which required emergency treatment but from which he recovered without incident. When Mr Pillay was more settled he was a little more forthcoming then previously. Following his previous admission to hospital he had struck up a relationship with a 24-year-old girl who suffered from a chronic and severe obsessive-compulsive disorder. He had met her on the ward. She was a shy, anxious girl whose psychological development had been disastrously interrupted by her severe symptoms and long periods of hospitalization from the age of 16. Mr Pillay said they had become engaged but then, after going to the cinema together and seeing a film with a strong sexual content, his fiancé had broken off their relationship. This was about six weeks before his admission and he had been drinking a bottle of vodka per day since then. Mr Pillay did not express anger towards his ex-fiancé but to a girlfriend of hers, also a patient, whom he accused of being jealous and at the same time prejudiced against him because he was an immigrant. Mr Pillay also talked of being lonely and of his friends being heavy drinkers. He had lost contact with those who were not. He was also seeing much less of his sister.

During this admission Mr Pillay was considered to be significantly depressed and he was treated with amitriptyline 50 mg three times a day. This had no effect on his mood. Just before his discharge from hospital after seven weeks as an in-patient, he was suspected of drinking again. He had no visitors during this admission.

Mr Pillay failed to attend for follow-up after his discharge. Within four months he was readmitted with delirium tremens ushered in by an epileptic fit. He was disorientated and had auditory and visual hallucinations. Shortly before he had been attacked and robbed in the street by some youths. Liver function tests were again abnormal (γ-GT 80 i.u./l). On neurological examinations there was a definite impairment of sensation below the mid-calf level and ankle jerks were absent. Clinical cognitive testing following recovery from the acute confusional state showed no abnormality. Detailed psychometry was not, however, performed. This time, after a period of 'drying out' he was referred to a day hospital. He attended for a month and joined in most of the prescribed activities although he mixed poorly with the other patients. Most sessions with the registrar responsible for his care were centred around his broken engagement which had had a profound effect on his already shaky self-confidence. During weekends at home he had no social support and he lapsed into drinking. He was encouraged to attend Alcoholics Anonymous meetings which he did only sporadically and another course of antidepressant medication failed to improve his mood. There were no signs of peripheral neuropathy on discharge and his γ-GT levels again fell to within normal range. When Mr Pillay finally returned to work he was informed that he would lose his job if his drinking continued. He moved out of his flat and took a room with a Mauritian family.

For three months following his discharge Mr Pillay attended regularly as an out-patient. He denied that he was drinking but it was strongly suspected that he was. He attended Alcoholics Anonymous irregularly. He was always polite and deferential in his manner but again revealed very little about himself. Nothing new emerged about his past life, nor was it ever clear what he was feeling during the sessions. He maintained that all was going well and he seemed to be gaining a measure of new support from the family with whom he was living. He contributed to the house by some redecorating and took some pride in this. An offer of antabuse for a trial period was rejected. He eventually lapsed from follow up again.

As predicted, Mr Pillay's drinking has continued with serious consequences. This situation creates a sense of hopelessness which may inhibit exploring other approaches. The reader should consider what potentially useful areas might have been ignored.

Reformulation

Diagnosis

Mr Pillay has continued to show dependence on alcohol with a series of syndromes of alcohol withdrawal—generally delirium tremens, but on his second admission an acute hallucinosis in clear consciousness. There has been a marked deterioration in his social functioning and his job has been threatened. A number of other complications of alcohol abuse have been present—liver damage, peripheral neuropathy and an episode of acute pancreatitis. They have so far proved reversible. The pattern of drinking seems to be one of intermittent spells of very heavy consumption interspersed with periods of more controlled, lesser consumption. This is probably why, despite many years of drinking, physical complications have not been more in evidence.

Aetiology

During the year or so since Mr Pillay first presented, there has been a great deal of evidence to confirm his social isolation and his difficulties in sustaining close relationships. No concern about him has ever been expressed to doctors by any friend or even his sister. He was never visited in hospital. He entered into a relationship with a young and very mentally disabled girl which looked doomed from the beginning. His expectation that it would result in a 'normal marriage' was grossly unrealistic. His reaction to her loss showed a marked sensitivity to rejection and in addition he was unable to perceive its origins in their relationship but instead blamed someone else. Mr Pillay has remained secretive and has failed to make a trusting relationship with a doctor.

Further investigations

It is striking that an informant has never been seen. At first, Mr Pillay refused but after this the issue seems to have been entirely lost. Had it been raised again it is possible that he might have relented and that his sister could have been interviewed. Some information might have been obtained which might have proved helpful in understanding why Mr Pillay was so concerned to avoid talking about himself and this might have suggested a better strategy for reaching him. The issue of an informant was probably lost because doctors had given up on him and because they sensed his likely embarrassment were certain facts to emerge.

The subject was a difficult one to broach with him and the cues he gave were to avoid it. It has meant, however, that he remains in many respects an enigma. A home visit could be organized by a social worker or community nurse. This might provide some useful information but it is unlikely that it will help to engage him in continued treatment.

Management

Mr Pillay has never stated unequivocally that he wishes to stop drinking. During his in-patient treatment he has transgressed the rules by slipping out for some alcohol. He has rejected the offer of antabuse. Antidepressant medication has not improved his mood state. A therapeutic alliance with the doctor has not been established. He attended Alcoholics Anonymous meetings sporadically.

At this stage the only option is to wait and see what happens. Mr Pillay has shown some inclination to return to the hospital when he becomes very ill and it is hoped he will return again when the need arises. Perhaps some new information will emerge or he will change his attitude. Considerable pressure should be exerted on him to allow an independent informant, such as his sister or a colleague, to be seen.

Referral to a specialist alcohol service needs to be considered if he returns.

Prognosis

This is very gloomy. It is likely that Mr Pillay will continue to drink, develop further physical and psychological complications and lose his job. His decline appears to be accelerating. Although there have been no intimations so far the possibility of suicide should be considered particularly if he were to lose his job. Perhaps a small hope resides in the support which he might be receiving from the family with whom he is now living.

Postscript

No more was heard of Mr Pillay for about nine months. He was then readmitted with the help of a work colleague, again with delirium tremens. His case notes regarding this admission were interspersed with many comments concerning his lack of motivation to stop drinking. No new points emerged in the history. However, he had managed to hold down his job and was still living with the same family. It was arranged for him to be seen at a specialist alcohol treatment unit where he was finally admitted. In the three years following this he never reappeared at his district hospital but it is known that he continued to hold his job.

6

A poor historian—the case of Mr David Stone, aged 55

Presenting complaint

Mr Stone was referred to the psychiatric out-patient department by his general practitioner who described him in his letter as 'forgetful and confused'. He attended with his mother, but they arrived at 6 p.m. and had to be seen by the emergency psychiatrist. Mr Stone was unable to explain why he was sent along to the out-patient department and the following account was therefore obtained from his mother.

She said that he had seemed very depressed for the last eight months, during which time he began to visit her every Sunday. When he came around he spent the whole day staring at the floor, muttering and saying very little. She had noticed that he ate very little and had lost a considerable amount of weight over this period. She attributed these changes to his poor accommodation, which was deteriorating as a result of a leaking roof. Although she had noticed these changes in Mr Stone becoming worse over the last eight months, she thought that his problems really began two to three years previously, when he was being divorced by his wife.

Family history

Mr Stone's father was a frequent gambler and heavy drinker. He often beat his wife and as a result of this she left him when Mr Stone was about five years old. Following this separation his father apparently suffered a 'nervous breakdown' as a result of which he was admitted to a psychiatric hospital. No further contact between him and the rest of the family ever took place. Mrs Stone remarried three years after separating from her first husband. She described her second husband as a 'very warm-

108

hearted, kind man', who seemed to get on well with all her family. He died suddenly of a stroke when Mr Stone was 18 years old.

Mr Stone's mother was 86 years old and presented herself as a capable, industrious lady. She continued to work as a cloth cutter until her late sixties. During her retirement she remained fully independent and maintained close contact with all her children, whom she saw frequently. In spite of her relative fitness and concern about her son's welfare, she said that she thought that she would be unable to take full responsibility for looking after him because of her increasing age and because he was becoming 'such a handful'.

Mr Stone had two older sisters. Mavis was 63 and a widow. She had been a successful student and matriculated at school. Two years previously she had retired from managing a grocery store. June was 58 and single. She continued to work part-time as a fabric buyer and lived with Mavis. The whole family lived within walking distance and maintained close and regular contact with each other.

Personal history

Mr Stone's birth and early development were normal. He attended school until the age of 14 and was considered an average scholar. While he was there he involved himself in numerous sporting activities and made plenty of friends. When he left school he was initially apprenticed to a plumber, but two years later he became a carpenter's mate. In 1943, when he was 18, he was conscripted into the Royal Navy and although he never saw active service, he spent eight months patrolling the North Sea in a motor torpedo boat. During his period in the Navy there had been one episode when he and some friends went absent without leave, as a result of which he spent three weeks in jail. He was never promoted and was demobbed in 1947, when he was 22 years old.

After he left the Navy Mr Stone had a variety of jobs, the longest of which lasted for 12 years, when he was a van driver. For the past five years he had worked part-time in an amusement arcade and as far as his mother was aware he had continued to do this on a fairly regular basis until his presentation to the hospital.

When he was 18 he married a girl he had known for six months, but this never developed into a stable relationship and his wife had several affairs while he was in the Royal Navy. This marriage ended in divorce when he was 23. During the next eight years he had several girlfriends, but never lived with, or became engaged to any of these. When he was 32, he married a 35-year-old Spanish lady whom he met while she was working as a waitress in London. She was a single parent with an 18-year-old daughter who lived in Spain. Mr Stone's mother always thought of her as the dominant partner in their relationship and often referred to her during the interview as a 'nagger'. The couple had twins within a year of marriage and the boy suffered a respiratory arrest when he was one year old, following an episode of pneumonia. He became mentally retarded and was designated educationally subnormal. As a result of this he was sent to remedial classes at school, but was never institutionalized.

Mrs Stone had decided to return to work when the twins were two years old, and Mr Stone's mother looked after them until they reached the age of 11. During this time the marriage steadily deteriorated. Mr and Mrs Stone had frequent rows about their son's welfare, her claims to independence and the extent to which she felt that his mother was attempting to organize their lives for them. These arguments became increasingly acrimonious and Mrs Stone continually accused him of 'turning out like his father'. As a result of these rows they separated and Mrs Stone took over complete responsibility for the twins' care when they were 11 years old. Their daughter eventually did well at school and passed three GCE A Levels, and their son moved from a school for the handicapped to a community day centre.

Following their separation Mr and Mrs Stone's relationship deteriorated and she divorced him three years before his referral to hospital. Since then he had no further contact with either his wife or his children.

Mr Stone had not generally been a regular or heavy drinker, but during the period surrounding his separation from his wife he frequently became drunk and abused her, both physically and verbally. His mother knew a few details of this episode but believed that it never led to any contact with the police. As far as she knew he drank very little alcohol at the present time.

Past medical history

Mr Stone received medical treatment for a perforated duodenal ulcer three years after he separated from his wife. He also suffered from a severe attack of 'bronchitis and asthma' which required in-patient treatment a year after this. Apart from these illnesses he had been physically fit all his life. He was taking no prescribed medication and was a non-smoker.

Past psychiatric history

Mr Stone was never seen by a psychiatrist before.

Previous personality

His mother said that he was always an easygoing, sociable person and that he had many friends who frequently sought his company.

Mental state examination

Appearance and general behaviour

Mr Stone was a tall, thin, handsome man who sat hunched up in his chair, staring at his feet. He made few gestures, apart from intermittently taking his reading glasses out of their case, putting them on, taking them off and then returning them to their case. He was casually but tidily dressed, appeared clean but had a noticeable growth of stubble on his chin.

Talk

Mr Stone said nothing except in response to direct questions when he would nod and say a few words before trailing off into mumble. For example, when he was asked if he had any problems he said 'I start to do something and . . .'. When he was prompted he said 'Well, um . . .'. When he did speak it was at a normal rate.

Mood

He looked miserable and his eyes frequently moistened, although he never actually cried. Occasionally he smiled in response to the interviewer's efforts to encourage him to speak.

Thought content

It was impossible to find out what Mr Stone was thinking because of his limited responses.

Abnormal beliefs and interpretation of events

None were elicited.

Abnormal experiences

None were elicited.

Cognitive state

Mr Stone knew the place and the year. However, he was unable to be more specific than this, despite prompting. When he was asked the date of the last war he replied 'I can't remember dates'. He was then asked to subtract seven from 100, but he remained silent.

Appraisal of illness

This could not be elicited.

Physical examination

A brief physical examination was carried out, which revealed no obvious abnormality except for evidence of weight loss.

Summary

Mr Stone is a middle-aged man who was brought to the psychiatric department by his mother. She said that over the last eight months he had become increasingly isolated, his mood had changed and he had lost a considerable amount of weight. She thought his behaviour had deteriorated over the last few years following his divorce and she described episodes of physical illness and heavy drinking which took place at that time. On examination he was miserable and showed poor concentration and memory. However, the most marked abnormality was his inability to initiate or maintain a conversation.

The unusualness of Mr Stone's presentation is worrying. Under these circumstances the formulation will be directed towards defining immediate management plans which will include the possibility of hospitalization and the organization of special investigations.

Formulation

Diagnosis

The changes described in Mr Stone, in the presence of his disturbed mood and cognition could be caused by either an affective illness of the depressed type or an organic dementing illness. The information available is insufficient to make a clear distinction between these alternatives, although depression would be a far more likely diagnosis than dementia in a 55-year-old man. However, there are certain features in Mr Stone's case which make a dementia more likely. Although he seems miserable, he does not demonstrate the severe manifestations of depression that would explain his near muteness. In particular, this appears to be a manifestation of his poverty of thought rather than a reflection of depressive retardation.

Aetiology

At this stage the relevance of aetiological factors to Mr Stone's condition depends upon whether they point towards a particular diagnosis or suggest fruitful lines of enquiry which might help clarify the diagnosis. For example, there is the possibility of an hereditary component since Mr Stone's father was also admitted to a psychiatric hospital. However, unless his father's diagnosis can be discovered this information is not helpful.

As far as the possibility of depression is concerned, Mr Stone's past history provides conflicting evidence about his vulnerability to psychiatric illness. He seems to have had considerable difficulties in establishing and maintaining long-term relationships with women and his separation from his second wife was associated with severe alcohol abuse and violent behaviour. These changes could be seen as a 'depressive equivalent' and would be consistent with his mother's suggestion that the final divorce from his wife had triggered off a 'depression'. On the other hand he has suffered from other severe stresses in his life—imprisonment for being absent without leave, a previous divorce, having a severely handicapped son—without any serious psychological complications.

If Mr Stone turns out to have a dementing illness it will be essential to consider all possible reversible causes, however unlikely these may be. These can be divided into the following: metabolic, which includes myxoedema, hypercalcaemia, vitamin B_{12} and folic acid deficiency and liver disease; infective, which includes syphilis or a cerebral abscess; traumatic, especially a chronic sub-dural haematoma, which might follow a relatively trivial head injury; finally, neoplastic, which can be primary or secondary.

Among these Mr Stone's history of drinking raises the suspicion of liver disease and his marked weight loss might have been associated with an underlying neoplasm.

The other major causes of dementia are parenchymal degeneration and cerebro-vascular, especially arteriosclerotic disease. Mr Stone's history of gradual deterioration without any step-wise episodes is more consistent with a parenchymal disorder such as Alzheimer's disease, which frequently occurs in this age group.

Further investigations

The major aim at this stage is to clarify the diagnosis. The most important aspect of this will therefore be a more detailed examination of Mr Stone's mental state, in particular an appraisal of his mood and cognitive functions. In addition to finding out whether Mr Stone has any depressive preoccupations, observations will need to be made of any variation in his mood, alteration in his sleep pattern or general evidence of retardation. He will also need a full and detailed examination of his cognitive skills which will include memory, orientation and concentration. An assessment of specific topographical cerebral functions should also be undertaken.

If it becomes clearer that Mr Stone is suffering from a depressive illness then it will be necessary to obtain more detail about its mode of onset and its relationship to his separation from his wife. However, should it become clearer that Mr Stone's illness is organic in nature then it will be important to find out whether he has suffered from any head injury, however trivial. In either case a detailed account of his drinking habits will need to be obtained.

Mr Stone presents one of those clinical situations in which a physical examination is imperative. Particular attention will have to be paid to any evidence of liver, cardiovascular or neurological disease, each which might be associated with a dementing illness. A bronchopulmonary neoplasm can also produce 'non-metastatic' effects similar to those found in Mr Stone and therefore needs to be excluded.

Special investigations are also required when investigating the possibility of a dementing illness. These are important not only to help reach a diagnosis, but also to exclude possible reversible causes of dementia. The routine investigations should include:

Full blood picture, serum B_{12} and serum folic acid;
Blood urea and electrolytes, liver function tests and thyroid function tests, serum calcium;
VDRL (specific tests for syphilis);
Chest X-ray and electrocardiogram;
Electroencephalogram (EEG), CT scan;

Management

Mr Stone should be admitted to hospital immediately because of the significant deterioration that has taken place in his level of function and the uncertainty surrounding his diagnosis. If he is found to have a depressive illness it will require urgent treatment. Furthermore, as an inpatient, it will be easier to undertake the essential investigations which in this case include detailed nursing observations of Mr Stone's behaviour and an assessment of his functional capacity on the ward.

Prognosis

This depends upon the diagnosis that is eventually made. If Mr Stone is found to be suffering from depression then this should respond well to appropriate treatment. However, if the diagnosis is a dementing illness then the outcome is poor, unless a reversible primary cause can be found.

Brief formulation

Mr Stone is a 55-year-old man who has changed from being an extraverted, cheerful person to one who is isolated and becoming increasingly miserable. On examination the most striking feature is his inability to initiate or maintain conversation.

Diagnosis

These changes could be explained by either an organic dementing illness or an affective illness, both of which could be associated with memory impairment, diminished concentration and a depressed affect. Although depression is more likely than dementia in a 55-year-old man, in Mr Stone's case there is little evidence that he is sufficiently depressed to explain his difficulty in maintaining a conversation, which presents itself as poverty of thought rather than depressive retardation.

Aetiology

Until a diagnosis is made the relevance of possible aetiological factors will remain unclear. Thus, if he is depressed, his history of a divorce, his long-standing difficulty in forming relationships with women and the emotional disturbance that followed his initial separation from his wife will all take on greater meaning. On the other hand if he is dementing this could could be due to a wide range of causes: cerebro-vascular, degenerative, neoplastic, metabolic, infective or traumatic.

Further investigations

It is essential to undertake a more detailed examination of Mr Stone's affective and cognitive functions. He requires a thorough physical examination concentrating on his cardio-vascular and neurological systems. Signs of any possible cancer or of liver disease should also be sought. A full range of special investigations needs to be undertaken concentrating on possible reversible causes of a dementing illness.

Management

Mr Stone should be admitted to hospital immediately, not only to obtain the further information, but because of the significant deterioration that has taken place in his level of function. If this is due to a depressive illness it will require urgent treatment.

Prognosis

If he has a depressive illness then this should respond to appropriate treatment. If however he has an organic dementing illness then the prognosis depends on whether a reversible cause is found.

Further information

Mr Stone was admitted to the ward. No further information was obtained from his mother about his recent deterioration and his ex-wife was not contacted. His mother insisted that he had only drunk heavily at the time of his separation from his ex-wife and confirmed that his deterioration had been a gradual one, with no sudden changes.

The nurses reported that he looked miserable constantly throughout the day although he did seem more cheerful when his relatives visited him. He slept well, attended regularly for meals, and ate all the food that was placed in front of him. He never spoke to other patients and ward staff unless they approached him and tended to remain isolated. On several occasions he left the ward, but he always returned unassisted before supper time. He dressed and undressed himself and knew how to find his own bed and the toilet. He was never incontinent.

Mental state examination (performed one week after admission)

Appearance and general behaviour

Mr Stone remained a rather dishevelled looking man. When interviewed he sat quite still and looked uncomfortable with a puzzled look on his face. He followed simple requests such as to take off his jacket, or to undo his buttons.

Talk

He only spoke when spoken to and gave one-word answers to the questions that were put to him. There was no change from the example noted when he was admitted.

Mood

He looked miserable and seemed to be somewhat perplexed. When he was asked directly whether he felt unhappy and wanted to cry, he replied 'yes'. When he was asked whether he had ever considered suicide or had noted any change in his sleep or appetite he replied 'no'. These responses were not conveyed with any emotion.

Thought content

Despite continual prompting, he was unable to communicate any of his thoughts.

Abnormal beliefs and interpretation of events

None were elicited.

Abnormal experiences

None were elicited.

Cognitive state

General knowledge. When he was asked to name the Prime Minister Mr Stone gave the name of the leader of the opposition. He knew the Queen's name, but when asked the name of her husband he replied 'I don't know'. He remained silent or replied 'I don't know' when asked other questions about general events in the news.

Orientation. He knew the name of the town he lived in, but was only able to say he was in hospital after being prompted by being offered several alternatives: 'hospital, railway station, post office'. He named the year correctly, but replied 'I don't know' when asked to name the day and the month. When asked what time it was he replied 'after lunch' when it was 4 p.m. When he was asked to give his address, he remembered the name of the road, but said 'I can't remember' when asked the number of his house. He eventually gave the correct number when he was offered three alternatives.

Past memory. He remembered the year of his birth, but was unable to state the day and month in spite of prompting. When he was asked his age he replied '45' and repeated this answer. He correctly gave the age at which he had entered the Royal Navy, but when asked how old he was when he had left the Royal Navy he replied 'the 1940s'. On repeating this question he replied 'I don't know'.

Recent memory. He was able to repeat immediately the examining doctor's name, 'Dr Williams'. However, five minutes later he replied 'Mr Wilson'. When he was asked to repeat 'Mr Albert Smith, 24, Peace Road, Southampton', his immediate reply was '. . . Mr Albert . . .'. and he was unable to remember that he had been asked to remember the address five minutes ago.

Concentration. He counted up to 19 and stopped when requested to do so. He was then asked to subtract seven from 100 and replied 'one hundred . . .'. In spite of further prompting he was unable to get beyond this.

Simple arithmetic. When he was asked to add seven and four he replied 'I don't know' and in spite of prompting did not give an answer.

Object naming. He was able to name correctly 'glasses' and 'buckle'. However, he called a watch a 'digit', a watchstrap a 'hand', an ashtray 'to put cigarettes in' and a jacket a 'cloak'.

Picture copying and construction. Mr Stone was asked to copy several shapes and to fill in the numbers on a clock face drawn by the doctor (Fig. 1).

Appraisal of illness
This could not be elicited.

Physical examination

Physical examination revealed only evidence of weight loss. In particular, his cardio-vascular system was normal, his blood pressure was 120/80 and there were no carotid or cardiac bruits. He had no clinical evidence to suggest that he had a neoplasm.

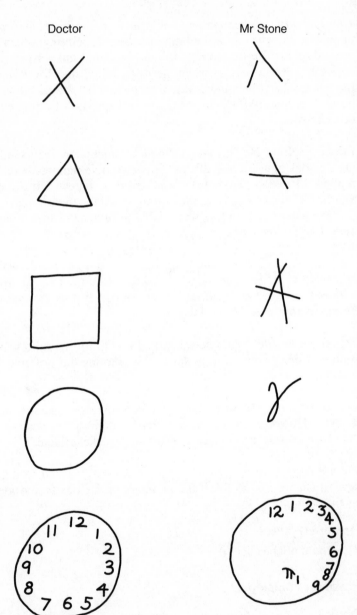

Fig. 1

A thorough examination of Mr Stone's nervous system indicated that it was also normal. In particular, the following features were noted. He was right handed and showed no evidence of right/left disorientation. He was able to take his jacket off and put it on again correctly. No abnormalities were found in his visual fields or his cranial nerves. Examination of his motor and sensory systems and of his reflexes was normal. No primitive reflexes (sucking, grasping) were elicited. There was no evidence that he ignored any parts of his body (anosognosia) and he showed no manifestations of astereognosis, agraphaesthesia, sensory extinction or visual inattention. Cerebellar functions were also normal.

All the special investigations were within normal limites, apart from the EEG and CT Scan.

EEG

'A bilateral abnormality is noted. The dominant frequency is slow and there is rhythmic theta activity over the frontal region. This latter feature is more evident on the left, but there are no focal features'.

CT head scan

'Moderately severe, widespread atrophic changes. No focal lesions seen'.

Sufficient information has now been gathered to clarify Mr Stone's diagnosis. We suggest the readers develop their own formulation before reading ours.

Reformulation

Diagnosis

The more detailed examination of Mr Stone's mental state has confirmed the severe impairment of his cognitive functions. He was more disorientated in time than in space, had a very poor grasp of general knowledge, a poor memory for past events, and an extremely distorted retention of recent events. His concentration was disturbed and he had acalculia. He also demonstrated a nominal dysphasia, a severe visuo-spatial agnosia, dysgraphia and his drawing of a clock face showed marked 'crowding'.

He continued to show poverty of speech and although he was miserable, there was a shallowness about his mood which also conveyed a sense of perplexity.

These features are consistent with a generalized cortical disturbance with particular loss of parietal lobe function. The generalized nature of this dysfunction has been confirmed by the EEG and his CT scan also shows signs of widespread cortical atrophy. These features are all consistent with a diagnosis of dementia of the Alzheimer type, which must be the most likely diagnosis, given the absence of any other primary cause. In particular, his mother confirmed that there had been no step-wise deterioration, which would have suggested a diagnosis of arteriosclerotic dementia.

The possibiity that Mr Stone's deterioration is secondary to an affective illness now seems very unlikely. No serious manifestations of depression have been observed by the nursing or medical staff and although he appeared miserable this was conveyed in a rather shallow fashion. The fact that he was perplexed is also consistent with a diagnosis of dementia. Although it remains possible that Mr Stone had a mild, coexisting affective disorder, this seems unlikely to have contributed significantly to his symptom, which all point to a significant organic deficit.

Aetiology

No new factors have emerged, although it is known that there may be a hereditary component to Alzheimer's dementia.

Further investigations

Since the diagnosis is confirmed it is now important to establish the level of independent function that Mr Stone will be able to sustain. A detailed occupational therapy report should be obtained and this should include an assessment of his ability to look after himself independently in his home accommodation. It may be that Mr Stone would be able to continue to live independently with support from his family and back-up from the social services, including meals-on-wheels and visits from a community psychiatric nurse.

His mother reported that his home had a leaking roof and so a thorough evaluation should be made of the quality of his accommodation and its suitability for someone in Mr Stone's condition.

At this stage it would also be useful to find out what Mr Stone does when he leaves the hospital.

Management

The main aim of management will be to maintain Mr Stone in the community as long as possible. This means that further assessments should be obtained as quickly as possible and appropriate social service support—home help, meals-on-wheels, community psychiatric nurse, day centre—should also be mobilized rapidly. Arrangements will also need to be made to maintain contact with him in the out-patient department. If Mr Stone is found to be capable of living independently then admission to a warden-controlled flat or an old age home may be necessary. At some time he may require admission to a psychogeriatric ward as his condition is almost certain to deteriorate.

It will be essential to keep Mr Stone's general practitioner fully informed of these details.

His family should be informed of the diagnosis and of its implications. They should also be consulted regarding the most appropriate way of providing support for Mr Stone in the community.

Prognosis

Alzheimer's disease has a poor long-term prognosis and 50 per cent of patients die within five years of the diagnosis being made. Features suggesting a worse outlook include an early age of onset, parietal lobe signs, and rapid deterioration. In the shorter term the prognosis may depend upon the presence of complicating factors such as depression. Mr Stone was functioning surprisingly well, considering the severity of his deficits. For example, he orientated himself well in the ward following his admission to hospital. He also had no features of depression. On the other hand his illness began when he was quite young and he seems to have deteriorated quite significantly over the last year. In the longer term, his prognosis is inevitably poor.

Postscript

Mr Stone was given a course of tricyclic antidepressants in order to see whether this would lead to any improvement in his mental state. In spite of a two month trial at a therapeutic dosage, no change was observed.

No functional assessment was made of Mr Stone, but it was thought on clinical grounds that he would be unable to maintain himself in the community. Mr Stone and his family were therefore advised that he should apply for residential care. Not only was his family unhappy about Mr Stone going into care, but there was a considerable delay in arranging for him to have an appropriate assessment.

Three months after he was admitted a nurse reported that she had seen him going into an amusement arcade, which was one mile away from the hospital, every day. This turned out to be his previous place of employment, and he was found to spend the whole day there sitting in a corner.

Following this discovery it was decided to try and support him at home and after discussion with his family, he was encouraged to spend several weekends at home, all of which passed without mishap. Four months after his admission he was discharged home and arrangements were made for out-patient attendance and regular social worker support. His family were advised to contact their local social services should the situation deteriorate.

Six months later Mr Stone failed to attend any of the out-patient appointments made for him and the hospital social worker was unable to contact him or his family.

7

A forensic problem—the case of Mr Loyola, aged 20

Presenting complaint

A telephone call was received from a solicitor, asking for a psychiatric opinion on Mr Loyola who had been charged on two counts of criminal damage, and one of grievous bodily harm. Having ascertained that it was possible to see his client and prepare a report in good time for his next hearing, the psychiatrist asked the solicitor to send a letter, setting out the points on which he wished to have an opinion, and copies of any statements in his possession. Copies of 12 statements, a list of two exhibits, a charge sheet with a list of previous convictions (all prepared by the police) and a copy of Mr Loyola's statement to his solicitor were accordingly sent with the letter.

The statements were of three kinds: by complainants, by expert witnesses (a doctor and a telephone engineer), and by Mr Loyola himself, under caution, to various police officers. Many of the statements were reports by different witnesses of the same incidents and, other than those of Mr Loyola, there was little variation between them. In fact they very often used exactly the same words. It was possible to build up a reasonable picture from them of the three alleged offences.

The first incident, leading to the charge of grievous bodily harm, occurred when Mr Loyola became involved in a feud between two families, the Porters and the Tanners. He, John Porter and one other youth went to Mr Tanner's home to exact retribution on one of its male members. Mr Loyola took the lead in this affair and got into an argument with Mrs Tanner on the doorstep which led to him hitting her twice with a hammer. The youths then ran off leaving Mrs Tanner lapsing into unconsciousness and covered in blood.

Four of the prosecution witnesses stated that Mr Loyola's

assault was unprovoked. Mr Loyola himself stated, under caution, that he had attempted to hit Mr Tanner, had been intercepted by Mrs Tanner who had kneed him in the groin, and that he had then 'cracked up' ('blacked out' to his solicitor) and 'started bashing away'. He was therefore pleading not guilty on the basis that he was defending himself against attack.

The second incident occurred about three weeks later when Mr Loyola had gone to the local social security office. He had asked to see a supervisor to request supplementary benefit, but he was told that, because of his previous aggressiveness, none of the staff would discuss this with him. The witnesses stated that Mr Loyola then began to shout, pulled a telephone off its wires and then punched a clerk in the stomach, 'very lightly' according to the clerk, before leaving. A telephone engineer confirmed that the wires had been ripped from the telephone and that the damage would cost £20 to repair. Mr Loyola intended to plead guilty to this offence, but described it as a 'joke'.

The third incident occurred when Mr Loyola was being questioned about the other two. He was put into a detention room although he later claimed that he had warned the police that he would 'crack up' if he was confined. Some time later a police officer returned to the room and found that Mr Loyola had gouged out pieces of the door, using the leg of a chair which he had broken. The officer reported that Mr Loyola had given the reason 'I just get so worked up'. Mr Loyola was pleading not guilty to this offence.

Mr Loyola had had 10 offences dealt with by Juvenile Courts between the ages of 14 and 16, including one for assault, several for carrying a weapon (a knife), and several for theft of motor cars. His only recorded previous conviction in an adult court was for driving whilst uninsured.

In his letter, the solicitor specifically asked about the following points:

1. Given that his client developed 'claustrophobia' in confined spaces and had done so when held by the police for questioning, should he be held not to be criminally responsible for his destructive behaviour whilst in the cell, and hence not guilty?
2. Could some other psychiatric reason be found to 'affect his criminal responsibility' for his other destructive behaviour (in which case his guilty plea might be reversed)?

3. Although psychiatric factors (his 'black-out') could not diminish his criminal responsibility for the grievous bodily harm charge ('but please confirm') could they be a mitigating factor, and should he be receiving treatment?

In the penultimate paragraph of his letter the solicitor expressed his concern about his client's fits of temper which could be 'extremely dangerous', and over the telephone the doctor was told that his client had stated that he would kill someone if he was sent to prison and so separated from his mother who, he said, relied on him.

An out-patient appointment was made, for which Mr Loyola arrived slightly early with another young man. Very unusually, the reception staff rang to ask that the doctor see Mr Loyola with the minimum of delay because he was causing a disturbance. In itself what he was doing—roaming round the waiting area verbally accosting other patients and staff and talking loudly and boastfully to his friend—was little enough, but the staff were frightened of him. The psychiatrist decided to see him in a room with an alarm button and near to the nurses' station, and to start the interview with a general account of his background.

Mr Loyola had no clear complaints. He would one moment say that he was perfectly well—'I'm no nutter'—and then say that his solicitor thought 'there must have been something wrong' for him to do what he did. He seemed to be in conflict about being thought to have any psychiatric problems; on the one hand the court might take a more lenient view if he had a psychiatric disorder, but on the other hand, he was unwilling to be considered in need of anyone's help.

The history was difficult to obtain although Mr Loyola became calmer when he was told that he could only be seen alone, not with his friend, and after the doctor had wondered aloud whether Mr Loyola's restlessness was an expression of his fear of psychiatric hospitals.

He eventually gave the following account.

Family history

Mr Loyola was the only child of a Spanish father aged 56 and an English mother aged 54. His father had been married and had children before leaving Spain to come to the United Kingdom but nothing was known of this family. As long as Mr Loyola had known him, his father had been a heavy drinker and had had an explosive temper. Mr Loyola remembered from an early age his father hitting his mother and hearing his unfounded accusations of her infidelity. In more recent times Mr Loyola and his father had come to blows. There had been several occasions during his childhood when his father had 'disappeared', for up to a year. Mr Loyola thought he had been living with other women during these periods. He had permanently left the family when Mr Loyola was 14. Mr Loyola had seen him occasionally at work in the subsequent two years, but he had not been heard of since.

Mr Loyola's mother had worked throughout his childhood and had usually been the breadwinner. Mr Loyola described her as a 'nervous wreck'. However Mr Loyola also described himself as being very close to his mother but 'hating his father'.

Personal history

Mr Loyola was born in hospital. He thought that his development had been normal and that he had been a healthy baby. He had lived throughout his life in a deprived area in a northern city. His mother had worked long hours when he was young and after school he had been cared for by an elderly neighbour, about whom he could now remember little. At the age of six he had been run over by a car whilst on a pedestrian crossing and suffered a head injury. Mr Loyola dated his tempers from this incident, and said that subsequently he had often been in trouble at school for violence. This was usually directed at members of staff but also sometimes at other boys, who teased him and called him 'fatty'. He was expelled from two schools for violence. On the second occasion, when he was 14, he described coming upon his headmaster leaning out of a sash window which Mr Loyola forcibly closed, trapping the man by the neck and then belabouring him with blows and kicks. Subsequently he failed to settle at two other schools, would not co-operate with a home tutor, and consequently failed to become proficient in either reading or writing. Mr Loyola worked for the council road maintenance department from 16 to 17 and a half, as did his father, but estimated that he had subsequently had about 30 jobs which had each ended after rows with his bosses. Currently he and a partner planned to set up their own painting and decorating business, having attended an evening class in 'do-it-yourself'. He would not discuss these plans and no assessment could be made of how realistic they were. Mr Loyola had always lived at home with his mother. He had no current regular girlfriend having just broken up, because she was getting too serious, with the girlfriend he had had since he was 16. Although Mr Loyola said that he had frequent sexual relationships he was unwilling to discuss these, or other aspects of his sexuality.

Mr Loyola was well known in his area, and did not lack for companions. However he appeared to have few, if any, close relationships, other than his stated closeness to his mother. Mr Loyola's main interests were his car and karate. He visited the gymnasium four days a week although the training programme had proved 'too much like hard work' for him to try and obtain a black belt. He was also a regular pub-goer and drank beer heavily on Friday and Saturday nights. He never drank alone, nor anywhere else but the pub, and had never experienced withdrawal symptoms. He had for a short while, about eighteen months before, used stimulants which he bought from 'mates at the pub' but had found that they made him too 'edgy'.

Mr Loyola had controlled the course of the interview so far, but futher relevant information had to be obtained by more direct questioning which it was likely he would experience as pressure on him. He had previously been very restless and the interviewer felt that there was a constant danger that he would suddenly walk out of the interview. It also seemed unlikely that Mr Loyola could be relied upon to attend a second interview.

It was therefore expedient to obtain the information which would enable the lawyer's questions to be answered as economically as possible. In order to do this, the interviewer decided to survey, in his mind, what he had observed of Mr Loyola's mental state, and then make a preliminary formulation.

Mental state examination

Appearance and behaviour

Mr Loyola was a plump, plain-looking man who looked younger than his age. He was rather restless throughout the interview, getting more so as it progressed.

Talk

His speech was rapid and loaded with swear words. He referred constantly to 'Paki-bashing', fights with 'the Bill' (the police) and his own physical strength and fighting ability. He said at one point to the interviewer 'I could easily take you on'. The form of his speech was normal.

Mood

Mr Loyola described himself as being depressed all the time and 'totally fed-up', but did not look sad.

Thought content

He was very worried about the possibility of going to prison.

Abnormal beliefs, and interpretation of events

None had been detected.

Abnormal experiences

None were alluded to, or apparent at the interview.

Cognitive state

His memory and concentration appeared to be good.

Summary

Mr Loyola is a 20-year-old inner city resident with an overworked mother who was probably usually too tired to be much of a parent to him, and a heavy drinking, quick-tempered father who never made an enduring relationship with either his wife or his son. He has had a history of temper tantrums stretching back into childhood when he had a head injury. He has been charged with three offences of violence about which his solicitors would like an opinion and the formulation will need to concentrate on these issues. Since there is a constant threat that the interview will end suddenly, the psychiatrist will have to decide whether Mr Loyola has a psychiatric illness.

Formulation

Diagnosis

The most immediate consideration is whether Mr Loyola's personality has changed recently. If so, this might indicate that Mr Loyola has developed a psychiatric illness. Mr Loyola has committed three offences within a short period and after a period of two years during which he has not been convicted of any offence. A change in his behaviour alone is a weak indication of disorder and may be due to a change in circumstances.

There are few symptoms and signs, independent of his behaviour, to suggest a psychiatric illness. There is no suggestion of a psychosis. Mr Loyola does complain of feeling depressed and also of panic in confined spaces. These symptoms, if they are recent, may indicate a depressive disorder, or an anxiety neurosis both of which may increase irritability, and predispose to violence. Mr Loyola is also a heavy drinker, and the possibility of alcohol dependence leading to chronic intoxication and consequent abnormally impulsive or explosive behaviour needs to be considered.

The next consideration is whether Mr Loyola has a personality disorder. This is a difficult judgement to make particularly in a patient who denies being in need of help but wants a court report and who may therefore give a very biased account of himself. Our experience has been that it is useful to consider three independent criteria, and that all of them should be satisfied if a diagnosis of personality disorder is to be made. There should be evidence of some particular socially deviant behaviour, or a cluster of related behaviours which are habitual and not under Mr Loyola's control. By itself, this may indicate only that Mr Loyola belongs to a sub-group whose culture admits of such behaviour. There should, therefore, also be evidence that these have adversely affected Mr Loyola's capacity to work or to gain satisfaction in social relationships and, finally, features of Mr Loyola's personality should correspond to common descriptions of personality disorder. This last criterion has the following advantages: it can be made more explicit than the second criterion, in some cases it suggests the presence of other symptoms or signs which can be searched for; and it may be helpful in guiding management. The information obtained so far suggests that all three criteria are likely to be met, but a diagnosis of personality disorder (the type of psychiatric disorder relevant to Mr Loyola's case) cannot be made until evidence of socially deviant (in Mr Loyola's case, aggressive) behaviour is obtained other than that which has led to the report being requested.

Two categories of personality disorder may be applicable to Mr Loyola. The first is personality disorder with asocial or anti-social manifestations. This would be consistent with Mr Loyola's lack of close relationships (although not his avowed close attach-ment to his mother), with his history in childhood of aggressive behaviour, and with his non-aggressive misbehaviour. However it excludes explosive personality disorder, a term best reserved for explosive outbursts which the affected person regrets and usually attempts, although often without success, to control.

Aetiology

Although it is too early to consider these in detail, certain factors suggest themselves for direct enquiry.

A closed head injury, such as Mr Loyola suffered at the age of six is associated with an increased risk of emotional or conduct disorders, especially irritability. These disorders may be the only detectable sequelae, or there may also be signs and symptoms of brain damage, possibly including epilepsy.

Brain damage in children may be the cause of persistent learn-ing difficulties leading to failure at school, itself a contributor to adolescent conduct disorder.

Epilepsy, especially temporal lobe epilepsy, is itself associated with irritability. 'Automatic' violence may occur during the state of clouding of consciousness pre-ictally, post-ictally or actually whilst paroxysmal electrical activity occurs in the brain. By definition this behaviour is not purposeful but onlookers may, rarely, have difficulty in appreciating the behavioural impair-ment. Irritability is also commoner in epileptic patients between fits, sometimes in association with mild electrophysiological dis-turbance which in some patients builds up over time until the epileptic threshold is reached.

Alcoholic intoxication is highly associated with all crimes of violence, but is particularly likely to predispose to outbursts in patients with a history of head injury.

Developmental factors contributing to a possible personality disorder are plentiful in Mr Loyola's history. Violent or antisocial behaviour in the father, neglect by the mother, serious marital or familial conflict, a lack of firm and consistent sanctions, poor relationships with peers, and problems at school are all associated with truancy, stealing and other conduct disorders in childhood and with personality disorder in adulthood.

Further investigations

Further information relevant to diagnosis needs to be obtained. Is there evidence of epilepsy? Is there evidence of irritability due to a specific, treatable disorder such as depression, or to a specific handicap such as brain damage? More information needs to be obtained about the incidents themselves, particularly about Mr Loyola's intentions and feelings beforehand, about his attitude now, and about the part played by disinhibiting factors such as alcohol, or bravado.

Further information about Mr Loyola's personality is also needed, particularly about its development, about his behaviour towards other people close to him, and about his interests and habits. There are also pointers to areas of enquiry relevant to management. First, Mr Loyola seems to have had many fewer convictions between the ages of 16 and 20 than he had between the ages of 14 and 16. Were there factors operating then which would be relevant to the prevention of offences in the future? Secondly, a probation order will almost certainly be one of the recommendations that the psychiatrist will consider. It is therefore worthwhile enquiring specifically whether Mr Loyola has been on probation, something which may not be apparent even from extensive prosecution statements, and, if so, how useful his relationship with a probation officer was to him. Three forensic questions which will affect sentencing have also been posed. Did claustrophobic panic affect his responsibility for the criminal damage? Is there any significance in his report of a 'black-out' when he committed the assault? Is his condition amenable to treatment?

In order to answer these questions, Mr Loyola's mother should be interviewed, and previous psychiatric records obtained, and the probation service contacted. Special investigations, such as

EEG should be considered when this other information is available.

Management

Although not enough information is available for a plan of long-term management to be made, the conduct of the rest of the interview is also an aspect of management. The most important consideration appears to be that Mr Loyola feels that his pride has been wounded by his coming to a psychiatrist. One way of reducing his anger about this (which might otherwise prompt him to cease to co-operate altogether) is to allow him to tell his story in his own way, and for the interviewer to reduce control over the progression of the interview to the minimum consistent with obtaining necessary information. It would also be important to balance lines of enquiry about his deficiencies, for example his difficulty in reading and writing, with opportunity for him to expatiate on his sources of self-esteem.

Prognosis

More information, as outlined above, is required in order to discuss this.

Further information

The interview with Mr Loyola was completed although he refused to attend again, either for a follow-up interview, or for an EEG. Mrs Loyola, his mother, was interviewed on another occasion. Although it proved that Mr Loyola had seen a psychiatrist on at least two previous occasions, the notes could not be obtained as the hospital where they were kept had been closed and the records destroyed. However, a psychiatrist who had seen Mr Loyola and his family when he was 12 was contacted, and remembered something of his impressions.

It was also discovered that the court had ordered psychiatric and social enquiry reports in relation to the grievous bodily harm charge. The psychiatric report was not forthcoming. Although Mr Loyola had attended to see the psychiatrist, the latter had failed to arrive within the half hour that Mr Loyola had been prepared to wait. However a copy of the social enquiry report was obtained. This further information, when collated, was as follows.

Family history

Mrs Loyola confirmed that Mr Loyola senior had been extremely violent, and also jealous. They had never married, and she was unsure whether her son knew of this. She said that as her son grew up, he had become increasingly like his father.

The offences

Mr Loyola thought that both of his acts of criminal damage were to some extent justified. In the case of the social security office, he felt that he had been unfairly treated, as the damage to the telephone was really too minor for consideration. He had no conception of the frightening effect of his rage on others. He also felt unrepentant for the damage to the detention room as he warned the police officer who took him to the room that he 'cracked up' in confined spaces, and because they had kept him waiting for an hour instead of the 20 minutes that they said. Mr Loyola had not been drinking before either of these incidents. Alcohol usually made him 'merry' and not irritable. He did feel that authority in general, and the police in particular, 'had it in for him'.

His assault on Mrs Tanner perturbed Mr Loyola more. He had not previously known the Tanner family, but was acquainted with one of the Porters. This man and his brother had seen Mr Loyola in a pub, and had told him four Tanners had attacked Mrs Porter and had asked him to help them 'sort it out'. He had replied 'I might as well'. On his way to the Tanners in his car he had stopped off at home to get a specially weighted length of wood, despite later claiming that he was not intending to fight but only to talk. Mr Loyola subsequently took the lead in the expedition and continued to do so even after the Porter brothers dropped out of the party. He told the psychiatrist that he would not have struck Mrs Tanner had she not hit him which, he stated, made him 'go blank and lash out'. He instructed his solicitor that he intended to plead 'not guilty' on grounds of self-defence for this reason. He remembered hitting Mrs Tanner and then running away to his car, which had been concealed. He said that afterwards he disposed of the length of wood by throwing it into someone's garden. He then went back to the pub, and then to a café where he got into a row with the owner and left without paying. Mr Loyola did not seem remorseful about the injury caused to Mrs Tanner, but did seem very frightened of going to prison. He said 'I'll kill anyone who sends me up'.

Personal history

School

Mr Loyola had first been suspended from school for biting and kicking at the age of five, shortly after his father had left his mother. His mother had not been concerned about her son's behaviour saying that it 'was a natural thing when they start school'. His education had subsequently been disrupted. He had failed to get into the Army because of his 'poor maths'.

Work

Mr Loyola had lost a labouring job which had lasted a month about one month before the incident with Mrs Tanner, and he had not worked since.

Forensic history

Mrs Loyola reported that her son had first been in trouble with the police at the age of 12. Although a list of Mr Loyola's previous offences was provided by the police, it emerged that this was incomplete and that several driving offences (connected with his continued use of his car after his licence had been suspended) were still outstanding.

Mr Loyola had been on probation for two years at the time of the offence. He had avoided contact with his probation officer, and resented his supervision. He did not feel that he had benefited from being on probation.

Previous medical and psychiatric history

Mr Loyola had been knocked down on a pedestrian crossing at the age of six and suffered a head injury as already mentioned.

Mr Loyola thought that he had been in hospital for one week after this and his mother thought that he had been unconscious for two days. Neither was absolutely sure. (It was too long in the past to assess his amnesia.) His mother had been awarded £150 compensation on his behalf. Suspension from school for misconduct made it impossible for any learning difficulty at school to be assessed, but he had learnt to read simple words as already noted.

Mr Loyola had never had a fit or a faint. He could remember no *déjà vu* experiences and had never been depersonalized or experienced derealization. He said that once his violence was 'set off' he did not know that he was doing it but could recall afterwards what had happened. His description was more like a description of losing control, rather than an alteration of consciousness.

Mr Loyola had first seen a psychiatrist at about the age of five, having been referred by the school because of aggression. He attended intermittently for several years and his mother was seen regularly.

At the age of 12 a psychiatrist made a domiciliary visit after Mr Loyola attempted to stab his father with a knife. Although there were no written records, this psychiatrist remembered finding the whole family 'very disturbed' and had offered family therapy which they did not accept. In fact, shortly after this Mr Loyola's father left the family.

For as long as he could remember, Mr Loyola had felt tense and angry when waiting or when being confined. He would not travel in tubes or buses for this reason. He was most comfortable driving in his own car, but even then had the windows down, even in winter. He disliked staying in one pub for any length of time, and could not sit through a film in a cinema. He could travel up to three floors in a lift but no more. Alcohol did not relieve these symptoms.

Mr Loyola was subject to overwhelming bouts of dysphoria, which he described as feeling 'empty'. These were worse when he stayed indoors or was alone for any length of time. They occurred once or twice a month. On these occasions he would shout at his mother, and had punched the walls, scattered cushions about, and, sometimes, smashed furniture. He disliked watching television but enjoyed trying to mend mechanical or electrical things. However, if his repairs did not go well he would get into a tantrum with frustration, and had smashed a television set, a stereo and a video-player at different times.

Mr Loyola had never felt sad or tearful but often felt empty and 'fed-up', as already noted. He had, he said, taken 'loads of overdoses', including one a month before the assault, 'because I have no money'. Usually the 'overdoses' were of his mother's diazepam. He had never had a definite intention to kill himself, and the 'overdoses' usually occurred during an episode of dysphoria. He had once jumped in front of a bus and, the day before the interview, had been playing with live detonators, one of which exploded, burning his hand.

Previous personality

Since childhood Mr Loyola had had an explosive temper which he made little attempt to control and which, in adolescence, had become incorporated into his ideal self which was as strong, powerful, and masculine. Mr Loyola could not distinguish anxiety from anger. His self-esteem was easily bruised and he blamed all his reverses on others. He was intolerant of all authority, such as the police, but he also tended to glorify the violent side of the latter's work. He was racially prejudiced and reported attacking immigrants ('niggers' and 'Pakis') both verbally and physically.

His mother said that he was 'easily led'. Mr Loyola had many acquaintances but no close friends. His mother described him as being very close to her but also reported that he had punched her on occasions.

Mr Loyola had had no close relationships with the possible exception of his mother and one girlfriend. He did, however, seem to attract male companions of his own age. Without constant companionship and activity he was subject to the bouts of dysphoria already mentioned.

Physical examination

This was not performed.

Mental state examination

Appearance, general behaviour, and talk
Already described.

Mood

Mr Loyola's predominant mood continued to appear to be one of tension rather than sadness or unhappiness. He denied ever having felt anxious or fearful. He had a long-standing difficulty in getting off to sleep, but did not wake early. His appetite was good although food did not 'taste of much' to him. There had been no recent change in his concentration, memory, energy, or libido.

Thought content

He was hopeful about his future, as long as he could avoid going to prison. Mr Loyola worried about prison, but did not otherwise ruminate.

Abnormal beliefs and interpretation of events

He had always been quick to assume that people were staring at him in the street or that casual remarks referred especially to him but was able to accept that he could not be sure that this was so. He was not deluded. He believed that he was well known to the police and that they victimized him.

Abnormal experiences

When asked about hallucinations Mr Loyola remembered that as a child he had heard a 'man's voice shouting', when there was nobody present and had thought he was 'going mad'. This had not recurred and he had had no other abnormal experiences.

Orientation
Normal.

Cognitive state

Attention and concentration. Good, despite his physical restlessness.

Memory. Good. His dating of events relating to the offences, for example, matched closely with that of the statements.

Intelligence. Mr Loyola's grasp and rapidity of thought suggested that he was of normal to superior intelligence.

Appraisal of illness

Mr Loyola did not consider himself ill, or likely to benefit from psychiatric care.

Now that the examination has been completed and his mother has been interviewed how should Mr Loyola's problems be formulated so as to answer the lawyer's questions?

Reformulation

Diagnosis

Mr Loyola lacks close social relationships and has failed to establish himself in steady work, despite over 30 attempts to do so, because of repeated uncontrolled explosions of rage. These have also led to his being banned from a social security office. He has failed to obtain a court-ordered psychiatric report because he refused to wait more than half an hour to see the psychiatrist.

Mr Loyola has had serious temper tantrums since he was five years old when they led to referral to a psychiatrist. They caused him to be suspended from school on at least two occasions, once after a serious and unprovoked attack on a headmaster when he trapped the man's head in a sash window and then kicked him repeatedly. Recently he has smashed valuable articles at home in temper, and also punched his mother. Mr Loyola's episodes of dysphoria may also be related to his tantrums since he usually, according to his mother, deals with them by trying to get into a quarrel with her. A possible connection may be that Mr Loyola feels 'empty' and 'fed-up' when frustrated but unable to attack someone or something else who is to blame.

There is also other evidence of repeated antisocial behaviour.

Mr Loyola regularly played truant from school, and had first been involved with the police at the age of 12. He had made many appearances in juvenile court for both theft and assault. Picking fights with 'Pakis' was one of Mr Loyola's main stated interests. He characteristically adopted a belligerent air with anyone whom he took to be an authority figure, as evinced by his behaviour during the interview.

Mr Loyola does not recognize that he has a problem with his behaviour nor is his antisocial behaviour entirely due to attacks of rage. 'Explosive personality disorder' is not, therefore, an applicable diagnosis but Mr Loyola does meet the criteria of personality disorder with asocial or antisocial manifestations. There is convincing evidence that Mr Loyola has a personality disorder since all three criteria of personality disorder are met: habitual undesirable behaviour (antisocial behaviour in Mr Loyola's case) leading to social dysfunction and characteristic of a recognized personality type.

Mr Loyola's personality is not so severely disordered, or the incidence of serious violence so frequent that the possibility of other contributory psychiatric factors can be excluded without further consideration. One candidate already considered in the initial formulation is epilepsy. However, both Mr Loyola and his mother stated that he had never had an unexplained fit or a faint. The violent episodes are not typical of either psychomotor seizures or epileptic automatism: Mr Loyola's behaviour is purposive during them rather than stereotyped, he has some memory of what happens, and he is capable of rational conversation during his outbursts.

Another possibility is that Mr Loyola has had an affective disorder which may have contributed to his instability and explosiveness.

Depression may be more difficult to diagnose in a patient with an antisocial personality. Some psychiatrists would extend the term widely to 'explain' antisocial behaviour. However, in preparing a report for the court it is wisest to base the diagnosis on such typical signs and symptoms of depressive disorder that there are, independent of the offence. Mr Loyola describes himself as 'depressed' and 'totally fed-up' and said he was so one month before the assault when he took an overdose. Mr Loyola has deliberately harmed himself on several previous occasions over many years. The experience of being 'fed-up' was usually short-lived although it may have become more prolonged since the offences, because of his fear of going to prison. He is not hopeless about the future, and has expansive plans to start his own business. He shows none of the 'biological' features of depression, his appetite is good, and weight steady. He does not wake early in the mornings. His concentration and memory are both unimpaired, and he is continuing with his usual interests. He can enjoy himself. A diagnosis of depression cannot therefore be sustained.

The possibility of anxiety state is suggested by Mr Loyola's dysphoria and his complaints of delay in getting off to sleep (a symptom often found in anxiety states, but not specific to them). Mr Loyola confuses anxiety and anger, making it difficult to assess whether his level of anxiety is pathological. However he does not experience his anger as 'suffering', he does not consider himself disabled by it, and he has no somatic symptoms such as palpitations or tremor. This makes the diagnosis of anxiety neurosis inappropriate.

Although Mr Loyola is not suffering from an affective disorder, it could still be argued that he was in a temporary state of unusual irritability. For example he could have been under unusual stress after losing his job. However, the diagnosis of personality disorder does not exclude such fluctuations, and the diagnosis of acute stress reaction or adjustment reaction is not appropriate because Mr Loyola's behaviour has not changed in kind (although it may have in intensity) as a result of the stress. Although Mr Loyola could not distinguish between anxiety and anger, he did distinguish panic from anger, describing it as 'cracking up' and was clear that this only occurred in specific situations, particularly confinement. Both Mr Loyola and his lawyer referred to this as claustrophobia. Mr Loyola's difficulty in using public transport, his avoidance of lifts and his avoidance of travelling in a car with the windows shut strongly suggest that he does have a significant disorder as they suggest. 'Claustrophobia' may be present alone as a specific phobia or may be part of a wider agoraphobic syndrome when it is associated with a fear of unfamiliar places or situations. This fear is often greater with greater distance from home and is reduced in company. it may be significant that Mr Loyola brought someone with him to travel across London to see the psychiatrist. Phobic neuroses of this kind are in our experience commoner in patients with antisocial personality disorder and may be often related to the need to feel constantly in control.

Aetiology

The aetiology of personality disorder is controversial. It is almost certainly multifactorial. The following factors have probably contributed in the case of Mr Loyola—neurological, imitative, developmental, social and contingent. Each of these suggest different management strategies.

Neurological

Mr Loyola's head injury in childhood may, if sufficiently serious, have left him with an increased tendency to attacks of rage. However, this cannot be the sole cause as explosiveness is only one aspect of Mr Loyola's violence, which anyway first began when he was five years old, before his head injury.

Imitative

Mrs Loyola felt that her son had become 'more and more' like her husband in his attitude and behaviour. This is unlikely to be attributable to heredity, which determines the transmission of much more elementary characteristics, but it can be explained by Mr Loyola's unconscious imitation of his father whose behaviour and temperament were very similar to Mr Loyola's own.

Developmental

Mr Loyola has never developed an inner world of feeling, and therefore has difficulty in reflecting on or modifying his immediate emotional responses. As a result Mr Loyola lacks inner resources of self-esteem, and therefore depends heavily on the esteem of others. This may be one explanation of the apparent contradiction between his view that his behaviour is simply a reaction to others, and other people's experiences of him as being very controlling. Not enough is known of Mr Loyola's early relationship with his mother to pinpoint the origins of these developmental difficulties although Mr Loyola was a 'latch-key' child from an early age, since Mrs Loyola returned to full-time work in his infancy.

Social

Mr Loyola's standing among his peers was apparently enhanced rather than damaged by his antisocial behaviour. It is noteworthy that the targets that he usually chose (such as immigrants and the police) could be seen as 'outgroups', upon whom assault might be more socially acceptable to his peers. Although this is not applicable to the present assault, it was committed during a vendetta between two feuding families, and Mr Loyola excused his involvement in it on the grounds that he was righting a wrong.

Contingent

It is often argued that violent behaviour is rewarded, and therefore sustained. However there is little evidence that Mr Loyola's behaviour is substantively rewarding. In fact, there are many occasions when Mr Loyola has suffered from his aggressive outbursts: for example when he has smashed valuable household items that would be expensive to replace, such as a television set or a video-recorder.

Three of the aetiological factors—social, developmental and imitative—are likely, on the basis of clinical experience, to be particularly important in the genesis of Mr Loyola's antisocial behaviour. Their relative importance can only be established by observing the effect of changing one or other of them during his future management. Some historical information about the effects of changed social expectations is available inasmuch as Mr Loyola's frequency of offences fell whilst he had a steady girlfriend.

Further investigations

A neurological examination and an EEG would be desirable, but Mr Loyola's refusal to re-attend precludes them. It is unlikely that a definite neurological abnormality would be found.

The attitudes of the probation services to a probation order should be discovered.

Management

If Mr Loyola was concerned to reduce his situational anxiety, it is likely that he could be considerably helped by a behavioural technique, such as desensitization or reciprocal inhibition. He is however, less likely to respond to a treatment based on 'relaxation' than someone whose fear of loss of control is not so great.

There is no simple treatment for Mr Loyola's personality disorder, but regular contact with a sympathetic and skilled professional may allow early detection of increased 'stress' and consequently reduce the likelihood of violence. However his personality is such that he easily feels slighted, is intolerant of frustration, and copes with many situations by exploding into a rage. The chances of developing a therapeutic alliance with Mr Loyola are therefore low.

Mr Loyola does appear to suffer from claustrophobia, or fear of being enclosed, to a moderate degree and this may have caused him to panic when enclosed in the detention room. Mr Loyola says that he damaged the door of the detention room in his desperate attempt to get out, and it is true that panic may lead to individuals with a phobia taking extreme steps to get out of the feared situation.

The solicitor also raised the question of Mr Loyola's plea. This is not usually a psychiatric matter but he may have been referring to Mr Loyola's 'intent'. This is a difficult and technical legal question rather than a psychiatric one. It is best to give the Court the relevant psychiatric evidence without further comment although, as there has been a suggestion of a 'black-out' which may suggest automatism to the court, the following statement could also be added. 'There is no evidence that Mr Loyola was unaware of the nature of his actions during any of the three incidents'.

The recommendations about treatment should mention the possibility of treatment as part of a probation order. But it should also be stated that the probation services must agree that an order is feasible. As it seems unlikely that Mr Loyola would attend even if psychiatric treatment was a condition of probation, a probation order cannot be recommended.

Mr Loyola might benefit from treatment, support and supervision but only on a voluntary basis, which, as already discussed, he is not prepared to accept. No specific recommendation about treatment can therefore be made to the Court.

Prognosis

Mr Loyola's prognosis will depend a great deal on his future social relationships. He may find a niche in a criminal fraternity, he may meet a strong, masculine but law-abiding figure whom he can imitate and then identify with, or he may continue to have difficulties in social relationships in which case he is likely to become increasingly vulnerable to depression or alcoholism with age.

Mr Loyola is likely to become less explosive with the passage of years but the risk of a repetition of serious violence will remain for some time in the future. A period of imprisonment seems likely either following the present offence, or in the future.

Brief reformulation

Mr Loyola is a 20-year-old unemployed Englishman, the son of an ill-tempered Spanish father and a hard-working English mother.

Diagnosis

Although Mr Loyola has bouts of dysphoria and has taken overdoses he has never had the specific symptoms of a psychiatric illness. However, there is independent evidence, mainly from his difficulties in social relationships, of a personality disorder which can best be diagnosed as a personality disorder with asocial and antisocial manifestations.

Mr Loyola also suffers from a moderately incapacitating degree of claustrophobia.

Aetiology

Several factors have contributed to his personality disorder. Particularly important are the examples of his explosive, and apparently selfish father, his failure to develop satisfactory 'inner objects' and the standing that his 'mean' reputation gives him on the streets of the inner city.

Management

In view of his past history of head injury more extensive neurological examination and an EEG are desirable, but not mandatory.

Since Mr Loyola does not and will not see himself as having or needing treatment no useful psychiatric treatment is possible. A probation order is unlikely to provide adequate supervision on past form. The court report should make clear the diagnosis, stress the absence of psychiatric illness, and point out that situational anxiety may have contributed to one of the offences.

Further investigations

A neurological examination and an EEG would be desirable.

Prognosis

There is a high risk of future violence which will slowly diminish with time. Mr Loyola is at risk of depression or alcoholism in the future. The outcome cannot be accurately predicted as it will depend to a large degree on the relationships that Mr Loyola forms in the future: continued poor relationships and legal problems, possibly leading to imprisonment, are likely.

Postscript

Shortly after a court report was completed, Mr Loyola was remanded in custody. His mother had telephoned the police during a row with her son, asking them to 'put him away'. Police officers had then gone to the house to interview Mr Loyola, who had attacked them. He had been arrested and charged with threatening behaviour.

Mr Loyola was subsequently sentenced to one year's Borstal treatment but, unfortunately, further details could not be obtained.

8

Fear of going out alone—
the case of Mrs Reiss, aged 48

Presenting complaint

Mrs Reiss, a 48-year-old married lady of Slovak origin, was referred to the psychiatric out-patient clinic by her general practitioner because of her fears of going out alone. These fears had been present for six years and for the past two years she had not ventured from her home unescorted. Attempts to go out alone resulted in panic and a fear of collapsing or dying. Mrs Reiss was somewhat better when driving a car, but she could not manage a journey lasting more than five minutes or so. Travelling on public transport was avoided, as were enclosed spaces such as lifts, the use of escalators and crowded, public places. The onset of these symptoms was described as sudden. Immediately following an argument with her husband, Mrs Reiss set out to post a letter but before she could reach the post-box she was overwhelmed with anxiety and dizziness and was forced to struggle back to her home. Her movements were drastically restricted after this episode but three years before presentation she improved considerably and for almost a year, although uneasy, she was relatively unrestricted in her movements.

However, her symptoms returned with even greater intensity two years before presentation and this followed the discovery that her sister had advanced carcinoma of the ovaries from which she died a few months later. The immediate precipitant of her relapse was again a row with her husband, after which she went out shopping, became panicky, and had to be brought home by a stranger.

Mrs Reiss said that she felt apprehensive before leaving her front door and after a few minutes in the street she would become panicky, dizzy, and sweaty and could feel her heart pounding. At this point she would turn back to avoid the development of a full-scale panic attack. When accompanied by her husband or by one of her children she felt uneasy but was able to enter crowded places for short periods of time. She could only shop in a small store and then only if accompanied. She could reach her restaurant, where she worked, from home only by car even though it was less than two miles away.

Mrs Reiss also complained of being depressed and of difficulties getting off to sleep. Two years previously she had developed hypertension and this was a major concern to her. Although her doctor had told her this was mild (BP 160/100) she could not be reassured. Another source of unhappiness was her weight. When she was 20 years old she weighed 48 kg but with the birth of each of her children and finally, following a hysterectomy four years previously, it continued to rise to its current level of 92 kg. Attempts to lose weight had been invariably unsuccessful.

Family history

Mrs Reiss came from a Slovakian Jewish family and lost both of her parents during the war when she was 14 years old. Her father was deported to an unknown destination while her mother and the children were taken to a concentration camp. There, her mother and three of her siblings were killed.

The family was a very religious one and she remembered her parents as being gentle and indulgent.

Two sisters and three brothers survived the war, Mrs Reiss being the youngest. Two years previously her elder sister died at the age of 66 of an ovarian carcinoma. Two brothers aged 59 and 56 were living in Australia. Both were happily married, but both suffered from hypertension. The remaining brother, who had lived in the United States, died eight months previously aged 49. He suffered from hypertension and developed 'water in the lungs'. Mrs Reiss last saw him two years previously.

There was no family history of mental illness.

Personal history

Mrs Reiss was born in a small town in Slovakia. Her birth and development were unremarkable and her memories of childhood were happy ones. She tended to be a reserved, shy girl but could not recall any special childhood fears. She recalled a marked sensitivity about menstruation as a girl. Her menarche occurred when she was 11 years old and her first period occurred while she was in the classroom. She felt extremely ashamed and feared returning to school until she was finally persuaded to do so after about a week.

As Mrs Reiss found it distressing to talk about her experiences during the war, these were not explored in any detail. However, references to the 'camps' cropped up frequently during the interview.

Almost immediately after the war, when she was 17 years old, she married a schoolteacher in her home town. She bore three daughters in four years, now aged 30, 29, and 27. Five years after her marriage, her husband died of meningitis at the age of 26. She was left with few supports, no close family, and worked as a shop assistant for the next five years.

At the age of 26 she managed, with considerable difficulty, to escape from Czechoslovakia and emigrated to Israel. There, she re-established contact with some distant relatives and worked on a kibbutz.

Three years later, aged 29, she married an Englishman, 15 years her senior and soon after they and her three children came to Manchester, England. They started a restaurant together which proved quite successful and in which she was working up to 18 hours a day at the time of her referral.

Mrs Reiss described her husband as a 'good husband and father' but made a number of references to his 'strictness' and 'unsteady' temperament. She said that he seemed to disapprove of many of her activities, such as driving a car. He also liked to have her near him even when this seemed unnecessary. Sexual relations had been infrequent for many years. Despite some quarrels she said that the marriage was a happy one. Mrs Reiss' children were all happily married and living in the same city.

Mrs Reiss said that she had very little free time. Her main pleasure was in seeing her grandchildren. She enjoyed listening to music and she was thinking of writing her biography. She rarely went out with her husband and she said that this was in part because of her fear of crowded places. A cinema, for example, was out of the question. Apart from the family, Mrs

Reiss had no close relationships. She said she had made no new friends since her marriage.

Past medical history

Four years previously, Mrs Reiss had a hysterectomy following investigation for menorrhagia. She did not know the reason. Two years previously, hypertension was diagnosed by her doctor, who prescribed propranolol 10 mg daily. She said her blood pressure had been 160/100.

Following the birth of each of her children and then her hysterectomy, Mrs Reiss' weight had risen without her ever being able to reduce it to its previous level. She attempted to diet most of the time, but stopped attending 'Weight Watchers' because she developed panic attacks when faced with a group of strangers.

Past psychiatric history

Mrs Reiss had never sought psychiatric help. Her doctor had, however, prescribed a variety of 'tranquillizers' none of which seemed to help. She had taken chlordiazepoxide for about nine months up until three months before coming to the clinic. She said that she was very sensitive to medication and readily experienced many side effects, particularly dizziness.

Previous personality

Mrs Reiss described herself as a 'quiet and sensitive' person who was upset by loud noises and particularly shouting. While being able to mix quite well with other people in a friendly but superficial manner she found it difficult, because of her reserved nature, to open up more and make deeper relationships. She preferred to keep her thoughts to herself. Most of her energies were put into her home and work.

Mental state examination

Appearance and general behaviour

Mrs Reiss was a moderately obese, well dressed, pleasant lady who found it difficult to talk about herself. She gave the impression that she was unused to doing so. She commented that it was unusual for her to show her feelings. On a number of occasions she was apologetic: 'I'm keeping you a long time, I'm sorry'.

Talk

She spoke with a strong European accent but her English was good.

Mood

During most of the interview Mrs Reiss did not appear especially dejected. She was animated when she talked about her children and grandchildren and she was able to laugh appropriately. On a number of occasions, however, her spirits sagged noticeably and she was on the point of tears. This was when she discussed the war, the death of her first husband, the death of her sister, and, most markedly, the death of her brother eight months ago. With regard to the last, there was no indication of any difficulty in accepting his death, of self-blame, of hostility or of an abnormal preoccupation with his loss. The intensity of her reaction did not appear unusually severe. This was also the case with regard to the death of her sister.

During the interview Mrs Reiss tended to be anxious and fidgety. She said she often felt tense and miserable but did not feel hopeless about the future. She said that 'one day everything will be OK'. Although she expressed a reluctance to 'bother the family' with her problems she was not self-reproachful. She had never entertained any suicidal ideas. There was some difficulty in getting off to sleep 'because my breathing is not right' but then she was usually able to sleep right through the night although she often had nightmares about the war. Mrs Reiss' appetite was normal and she was able to concentrate and function well at her work. Somatic symptoms of anxiety were only present when she faced going out on her own.

Thought content

Mrs Reiss described her fears of going out in considerable detail, but with little emotion.

An important theme that emerged during the interview was that of illness. Mrs Reiss worried a lot about illness in others and in herself. 'After the camps when you hear things, it's worse'.

Thinking about her raised blood pressure made her frightened and she found it difficult to accept that it was only mildly elevated. Unpleasant, though only momentary sensations in her head, she tended to attribute to her hypertension. Dizziness, in particular, was feared. She admitted to ruminating for long periods on her health and she made many visits to her general practitioner asking him for further tests. She said she was easily fatigued and had to force herself to keep going.

Abnormal beliefs and interpretation of events
None were elicited.

Abnormal experiences
None were elicited.

Cognitive state
There were no abnormalities on cognitive testing.

Appraisal of illness
Mrs Reiss said she needed help with her fears and expressed the hope which she half-recognized as unrealistic, that there might be a tablet which could remove them. She was reluctant to commit herself to a course of treatment without knowing all the details first and said she might have difficulty in getting time off work.

Physical examination

This was not performed apart from taking her blood pressure. This was 160/90.

Interview with informant

Mrs Reiss was accompanied by her daughter. The history as given by Mrs Reiss was confirmed in all its essential points.

The patient was described by her daughter as a person who tended to worry excessively and who was easily upset by displays of temper in others, by illness and death (even in people she did not know well) and by any reference to war. However, she was also capable of stubborn determination particularly in her management of the business. Rarely had Mrs Reiss revealed her innermost feelings to anyone in the family, although her loyalty to them was unstinting. Mrs Reiss had rarely talked about her wartime experiences and she could not be drawn into discussion about her life during this period. To others she invariably gave the impression of being a friendly and cheerful but 'aloof' person.

The daughter described the marriage between her mother and stepfather as a good one. She said her stepfather could be rather rigid in his views and was often temperamental. At these times her mother retreated and arguments were never sustained. Mr Reiss was unable to understand his wife's symptoms but seemed to accept them with little irritation. Mrs Reiss had virtually no social life outside her immediate family.

Mrs Reiss was very distressed after the deaths of her sister and then her brother, but she surprised her daughter with the apparent normality of her grieving.

Summary

Mrs Reiss presents with a six year history of fears of going out alone as well as some more specific fears of enclosed spaces and of escalators. She complains also of feeling miserable, of being overweight, and of the state of her physical health.

However, these problems are overshadowed by the implied enormity of her experiences as a concentration camp victim. In the formulation it will be important to consider how these experiences might be related to her current condition neither using them as a blanket explanation nor ignoring them totally.

Formulation

Diagnosis

The syndrome presented by Mrs Reiss is that of agoraphobia. Most of the typical features are present including extreme anxiety if she should leave her home or another 'secure' place unaccompanied. Public or crowded places are particularly feared. She has been virtually housebound for the past two years and is only able to venture out in the company of a trusted friend. Her fears are irrational, grossly disproportionate, and they lead to avoidance of the feared situation(s). More specific fears, like those she described of escalators, are also common in patients with this condition, as are experiences of depersonalization.

The major differential diagnosis in this case is between agoraphobia as a primary disorder and its development secondary to a depressive illness. The relationship between agoraphobic symptoms and depressed mood is complex. Depressive symptoms not amounting to a depressive illness are common in patients with agoraphobia. However, agoraphobic symptoms may appear for the first time in the context of a primary depressive illness. In these cases the typical symptoms of a depressive illness would be apparent. The agoraphobic symptoms follow the natural history of the underlying illness and usually remit when the depression does. The course is therefore likely to be one of a single episode lasting six to nine months or an episodic one with recovery between fairly clear-cut relapses.

In Mrs Reiss' case there is an absence of typical depressive symptoms, such as guilt, hopelessness, or diurnal variation of mood. There is also the long duration of the agoraphobic syndrome, notwithstanding a fairly long period of partial remission. These points argue strongly against a primary diagnosis of depressive illness.

An atypical feature in Mrs Reiss' case, is the relatively late onset of her agoraphobic symptoms when she was aged 42 years. Agoraphobia as a primary disorder usually commences before the age of 35 years.

Another notable aspect of Mrs Reiss' presentation is her preoccupation with her physical health. Although in part understandable in view of her strong family history of hypertension, her concerns with her blood pressure seem excessive and could be termed 'hypochondriacal'. They appear disproportionate to her mildly elevated blood pressure, they are associated with an unusual attention to physical sensations and she cannot be reassured as to their true nature.

The agoraphobia does not, in Mrs Reiss' case, appear in the setting of prominent anxiety symptoms outside the feared situations. Her tendency to worry excessively is a personality characteristic rather than a new development suggesting a morbid process.

There are also two physical diagnoses, obesity and hypertension. Mrs Reiss is clearly substantially above the mean weight for someone of her age and although her blood pressure was normal in the clinic it had been raised on a number of occasions when she consulted her general practitioner.

Aetiology

Mrs Reiss has had a life of extraordinary pain and misfortune. Although it is tempting to attribute all her difficulties to this, an attempt should be made to link her problems more specifically to particular antecedents.

An outstanding feature of Mrs Reiss' history is her wartime experience involving losses in her family and incarceration in a concentration camp. People who have survived this exposure to overwhelming fear, grotesque deaths, helplessness, physical abuse, and dehumanization are often left with a number of special vulnerabilities, and Mrs Reiss gives evidence of some of these. She has an indelible 'death imprint' which has sensitized her to illness and death in relatives and friends. This was probably due to the impossibility of mourning her dead relatives in the midst of an appalling struggle for survival. Her experience of devastating loss of life, family, and community are associated with a basic insecurity, a lack of social belongingness, and the loss of a sense of continuity with the past. After the war Mrs Reiss married quickly and it is easy to imagine how important it must have been for her to create anew, a family life. Her first husband then died, again in circumstances when mourning must have been difficult, due this time to the needs of her young children and the requirement to press on in difficult times. Mrs Reiss' movements between different countries and the absence of a stable home must have also contributed to a sense of rootlessness and it is noteworthy that her symptoms have the effect of keeping her in one 'secure' place, her home.

It is in this context that Mrs Reiss' present relationship with her husband must be considered. A strong and stable family unit is especially important to her. She has no close relationships outside her family, not in itself surprising in someone who has experienced so much hostility in the world and who might thus have a pervasive difficulty in trusting 'outsiders'. Although Mrs Reiss said that her marriage was a good one she described sensitivity to her husband's outbreaks of temper. A direct precipitant of her illness was a quarrel with her husband and a major exacerbation after a period of improvement again followed directly after another quarrel with him. One senses that Mrs Reiss' loyalty to her family is such that she is unlikely to speak critically of them to an outsider and that her family is so crucial to her sense of security that she would be likely to tolerate much from her husband that was not to her liking. It is perhaps surprising that Mr Reiss did not accompany his wife to the hospital in view of the long history and the handicapping nature of her disorder.

Of more recent events in Mrs Reiss' life, the deaths of first her sister and then her brother, stand out. Bearing in mind Mrs Reiss' sensitivity to illness and death it does not come as a surprise that her agoraphobic symptoms emerged more intensely following her sister's illness and death. One might have expected to find evidence of a morbid grief reaction following these deaths but this seems not to have been the case. She is sad about these losses but appears to have come to terms with them. The development of hypertension also coincided with the exacerbation of Mrs Reiss' symptoms and is likely to have acted as yet another stressful experience.

Overall, then, a number of Mrs Reiss' past life experiences can be seen as shaping a predisposition to some kind of psychological disorder as well as possibly exacerbating and maintaining one. However, why it should have taken the form of an agoraphobic syndrome is not fully explicable in these terms. In Mrs Reiss' case we do not have the benefit of a full family history which might have revealed similar problems in other members. Mrs Reiss' sensitivity to her menarche and her anxiety about going to school suggest that she was a rather anxious child, but this is tentative. A past history of school refusal and of undue separation anxiety is common in patients with agoraphobia.

Mrs Reiss' phobic symptoms can be seen more directly as the outcome of a learning process. Fears can be learnt as a response to previously neutral stimuli by 'classical' conditioning. This is most readily apparent for simple fears of specific objects. However, generalization from the initial stimuli may occur and here an important role can be ascribed to the symbolic associations of the stimuli for the individual. This type of learning is enhanced when the subject is anxious or distressed. In Mrs Reiss' case, the initial fear reaction occurred when she was in the street alone where multiple stimuli were available for association. Symbolic meanings for her, of crowded places and being alone could have related to past experiences of crowded camps. Whatever the process of the learning involved, an important mechanism in perpetuating the fear (its failure to 'extinguish' with time) is the avoidance of the feared situation. By leading to a reduction in anxiety, avoidance, in fact, reinforces the fear.

Some understanding of Mrs Reiss' hypochondriacal preoccupations can be gained from the history. There is a strong family history of hypertension leading, in her brother's case, to death. The physical abuses experienced by concentration camp inmates may be associated with later concerns over bodily integrity and the fear of permanent damage. There may be some confusion in Mrs Reiss' mind between the sensations of 'dizziness' which she attributes to her hypertension and the 'dizziness' which she experiences during episodes of anxiety which serve to intensify her self-absorption in her physical state. Her sensitivity to the 'side-effects' of tablets may also reflect her heightened vigilance to somatic sensations.

Mrs Reiss' obesity seems linked to a combination of weight increase with age and particularly in response to childbirth and hysterectomy. It is not the juvenile onset type where constitutional factors play a more important role. Past experience of starvation during the war might have contributed by creating a special preoccupation with food and through the association of thinness with suffering. Mrs Reiss' work as a caterer means that she is constantly exposed to food and this makes dietary restriction very difficult.

Further investigations

Although sufficient information has been obtained for a diagnosis to be made, before treatment can proceed a more detailed account is necessary of Mrs Reiss' fears and the limitations which they place on her. A clinical psychologist is experienced in making such an assessment and could propose a systematic treatment strategy based on learning theory principles.

It is not clear why Mrs Reiss, in view of the chronicity of her illness, has presented for help at this particular time. It is possible that a recent change in her circumstances, such as her marriage, has upset a pre-existing balance.

We do not know Mr Reiss' attitude to her symptoms although he must have been affected by them. Mr Reiss may need to be involved in treatment either in a general encouraging role or more directly in supervising her treatment activities. If there are important tensions in the marriage which contribute to Mrs Reiss' illness it might prove valuable to have some joint sessions. Mr Reiss thus needs to be seen both as an informant and to assess his willingness to be involved in the treatment.

Mrs Reiss' general practitioner should be consulted for further information about her hypertension and also about the treatment he has offered for her fears and her response to it. The precise reason for Mrs Reiss' hysterectomy is worth ascertaining as in someone with hypochondriacal concerns it may turn out to have been the result of persistent requests for help rather than of clear indications for surgery.

Management

Two alternative psychological methods should be considered, as well as the possibility of medication.

The first approach is supportive psychotherapy. The aim would be to establish a special type of 'working relationship' with Mrs Reiss in which she would find support and some advice in her endeavours to overcome her disabilities. Factors which have contributed to her illness could be explored with her in the context of a safe and trusting relationship with the therapist. Improvement would be predicted as the result of Mrs Reiss' acquisition of an understanding of her symptoms as arising from the operation of psychological influences, together with the therapist's encouragement to extend her range of activities in feared situations. The focus of treatment would not be primarily on her symptoms but on the psychological mechanisms she employs in dealing with such problems as illness, death, and losses.

The second method, systematic desensitization, would focus more directly on Mrs Reiss' symptoms, assuming them to be a learnt, maladaptive response to situations which are reinforced by avoidance. The principles involved are regarded as the same as those involved in normal learning and these principles are applied in the treatment as well. The situations which Mrs Reiss fears would be carefully delineated as would her usual behavioural responses to them. Treatment would require that she change her behaviour in the feared situations and this would depend on exposure to those situations rather than avoidance. A strategy of exposure could be planned, usually in a series of graded steps representing a hierarchy of situations, increasing in their fear-inducing qualities as perceived by the patient. Mrs Reiss would then be encouraged to work through this hierarchy, progressing to the next step on the hierarchy when she is able to feel relaxed at the previous one. Relaxation exercises might prove helpful here. It is anticipated that her fears will become extinguished as avoidance is overcome and she learns that catastrophe does not ensue from exposure. In theory the relationship with the therapist would be different with this approach, in that he or she would be more didactic and less concerned with discovering 'psychological meanings'.

Although in practice there is considerable overlap between these strategies there is a good reason in Mrs Reiss' case for emphasizing a behavioural approach. Given her past experience and the observations made during her interview, it is likely that she will find it difficult to make the sort of trusting relationship with a stranger in which she will feel comfortable in disclosing her inner feelings and in discussing the powerful experiences in her past. Her co-operation is more likely to be gained with an approach which is more directly linked to her presenting complaints. The treatment can be carried out by a psychiatrist or a clinical psychologist in the out-patient department.

An antidepressant can be helpful when depressive features are prominent. Although in Mrs Reiss' case there is no indication for this at present, it is worth bearing in mind for the future as an adjunctive measure.

In some patients even when depression is not prominent, panic attacks and phobic symptoms may be helped by a tricyclic antidepressant or by an MAO inibitor, although improvement usually requires a number of months of treatment. Benzodiazepines may also be of value in reducing anxiety if taken before the patient enters her feared situations. However, this does not generally help the patient to overcome her fears when she is not on medication.

In Mrs Reiss' case, where a long history is in evidence, a more direct attack on her symptoms is preferable to a palliative approach with benzodiazepines. There are two further worries about prescribing a benzodiazepine in her case. First, she is very sensitive to the unwanted effects of medication and these may make her even more preoccupied with her physical state and secondly, because of the chronicity of her fears, she may become dependent. A trial of a tryicyclic antidepressant or an MAO inhibitor could be held in reserve if a behavioural-psychothera-peutic approach fails to bring about an improvement.

Mrs Reiss' blood pressure needs to be monitored and at present propranolol, although in small dosage, seems adequate to control it. Propranolol also has a direct anxiety-reducing effect but usually at a higher dosage.

At this stage Mrs Reiss' hypochondriacal concerns and her obesity are not the most important issues. If her anxiety can be reduced, her hypochondriacal fears may lessen also. The treat-ment of obesity is difficult at the best of times and this could be left for review at a later stage if she overcomes her fears of going out alone.

Prognosis

As Mrs Reiss' agoraphobic symptoms have been present for six years, the chances of a complete and permanent recovery from these is slight. A full recovery with this condition is most likely when the symptoms have been present for less than a year.

However, of importance in assessing the prognosis is Mrs Reiss' pre-morbid adjustment. Although her life has been an extremely difficult one she has been able to make a good adjust-ment in a number of respects. Despite the loss of her first husband, for example, she has managed to make a second and durable marriage. Much determination has been shown by her in overcoming major crises in the past. Her ability to work has remained unimpaired. These personality strengths are important in preventing the development of the even more severe restric-tion of activities which may occur with this disorder.

Mrs Reiss' willingness to become involved in treatment may be an important contributor to the eventual outcome. Her motivation for change is a little doubtful, particularly as she has delayed her request for help for such a long time.

Overall, it seems likely that Mrs Reiss will continue to function socially at a reasonable level, but that unless she works very hard with her treatment, her symptoms will persist to a variable degree. The severity of her symptoms is likely to depend on the occurrence of significant life events to which she is particularly vulnerable—loss, illness, and death. These are likely to lead to exacerbation.

Brief formulation

Mrs Reiss presents with a six-year history of fear of going out alone as well as some more specific fears of enclosed places and of escalators. She complains also of feeling miserable, of being overweight and of the state of her physical health.

Diagnosis

Mrs Reiss presents with the syndrome of agoraphobia. Most of the typical features are present. The major differential diagnosis is of agoraphobia as a primary disorder or of its development secondary to a primary depressive illness. The former is favoured by the long duration of the symptoms and the absence of prominent depressive symptoms. The patient also expresses some hypochondriacal preoccupations most marked since the development of hypertension two years ago. These appear to be founded on an anxious personality. She is also moderately obese and has hypertension.

Aetiology

Mrs Reiss has had a life of extraordinary misfortune. She lost most of her family during the war and was herself incarcerated in a concentration camp. Shortly after the war she also lost her first husband. A stable family unit is extremely important to her but there is a suggestion of difficulties in her relationship with her second husband.

More recently she has lost two siblings and the death of her sister two years ago was associated with a marked exacerbation of her symptoms. She also developed hypertension at that time which probably also aggravated her agoraphobia as well as intensifying her hypochondriacal preoccupations. A strong family history of hypertension is also important here.

There is some evidence that she was an anxious child and experienced undue separation anxiety at school.

Whatever the processes of learning involved in her agoraphobic symptoms, her avoidance of the feared situations has reinforced them.

Further investigations

A more systematic assessment of Mrs Reiss' fears and her responses to them is necessary. It is not clear why she has presented at this time after a six-year history. Her life situation at the onset of the symptoms as well as her marital relationship need further exploration. Mr Reiss should be seen. Her general practitioner should be asked to provide information concerning her past medical and psychiatric history.

Management

There are two broad options—supportive psychotherapy aimed at elucidating the psychological mechanisms involved in her symptoms or a behavioural approach such as systematic desensitization. It is essential that she should be exposed to the feared situations to overcome the reinforcement of her fears. A good relationship with the therapist will be essential. A number of considerations would commend a behavioural emphasis in Mrs Reiss' case.

There is no indication for medication at present but a trial of an antidepressant drug may be held in reserve. At this stage her hypochondriacal preoccupations and her obesity are not the most important issues. It is hoped that if her general level of anxiety is reduced, the former will become less intrusive.

Prognosis

The likelihood of a complete and permanent recovery after six years of illness is slight. However, Mrs Reiss has important personal resources which are manifest through her history which suggest that she will continue to function socially at a reasonable level and which could support her endeavours to improve. Her motivation for change is, however, a little doubtful.

Further information

Mrs Reiss was seen by a clinical psychologist. Her daughter accompanied her as Mr Reiss was away in the United States on a business trip.

The psychologist's report was as follows:

A detailed assessment of Mrs Reiss' fears was made. There are two categories of situations which are anxiety provoking:

(*a*) distance from home (or safe place) alone;
(*b*) situations associated with looking up or down (e.g. escalators in tube stations).

Situations inducing the highest self-ratings of fear on a 0–5 scale are:

(*i*)   shopping in the local shopping centre;
(*ii*)   walking more than 15 minutes from home;
(*iii*) a bus journey of more than 15 minutes;
(*iv*)   travelling on the underground;
(*v*)   using an escalator.

Situations giving lesser difficulty (rated 2–3) include crossing a main road, shopping in a local shop, sitting in a cinema, visiting the synagogue and driving more than five minutes from home.

Fear is diminished by being accompanied by a trusted person, using a shopping trolley, darkness, having a way open for a quick return home and thinking about something else (especially her grandchildren). Her fear is made worse by arguments with her husband, hearing bad news especially concerning illness or death, and having to cross a main road.

At present she cannot walk unaccompanied more than three houses from her own home but she can drive for five minutes before having to turn back.

The role of Mrs Reiss' husband was discussed and her daughter provided some useful information about this. Mr Reiss has contradictory views about the problem. On the one hand he usually behaves as if the problem does not exist or that it is simply a matter of will-power; on the other hand he often maintains that if his wife has this problem then she should not drive, go out, etc. To some extent at least he appears to be contributing to the problem by discouraging her from going out, thus reinforcing her avoidance of feared situations.

The clinical psychologist also explored further the circumstances surrounding the onset of the disorder. This time Mrs Reiss said that her symptoms first began when her husband and she quarrelled on the way home from an enjoyable evening out with a group of friends. A few months before this, Mrs Reiss' daughter had left home after getting married, being the last of her children to do so.

When treatment was discussed, Mrs Reiss seemed surprisingly reluctant to embark on this but after some discussion with her daughter she agreed to 'give it a try'.

The general practitioner provided some further information in response to a letter from the psychiatrist. Mrs Reiss' blood pressure was first noted to be elevated two years ago and had on a number of occasions been 160/105. With medication it was well controlled but Mrs Reiss was not able to be reassured about this. The general practitioner had not been aware of the full extent of Mrs Reiss' phobic symptoms although he recognized that she had suffered from 'anxiety for many years'. Chlordiazepoxide 10 mg twice a day had been prescribed for about nine months but this did not prove helpful. The hysterectomy had been performed for persistent menorrhagia caused by fibroids.

Having received the psychologist's report the psychiatrist is in a position to start treatment. At this stage the reader should consider whether the original plan needs to be modified.

Reformulation

Diagnosis

As above.

Aetiology

Some important new points have emerged. Mr Reiss' attitude to Mrs Reiss' disorder is problematical and he expresses ambivalent feelings about it. His behaviour appears to encourage the maintenance of her symptoms. A new version of the onset of Mrs Reiss' symptoms again places it in the context of a quarrel with her husband. Her daughter's leaving home is very likely to have been, in part, a sad experience for Mrs Reiss as her family is so important to her. It also meant that she was now alone with her husband and probably left to confront problems with him more directly. However, it is still unclear why Mrs Reiss presented at this time.

Further investigations

It will be important to assess Mr Reiss' attitude at first hand.

Management

A behavioural strategy has been offered by the psychologist to be carried through by her.

This involves a programme of graded pactice involving practice sessions in the hospital and prescribed daily 'homework'. A hierarchy of fearful situations in ascending order of anxiety was constructed with her help and at each hospital session homework for the intervening period is to be planned involving narrower hierarchies. For the first session this involves walking for even greater distances from home, each time up to a point where anxiety is manageable. Mrs Reiss will be instructed to keep a diary of all of her outings and to record the distance travelled and anxiety experienced.

Prognosis

Mrs Reiss' questionable motivation and Mr Reiss' apparent ambivalence might prove important limitations on progress.

Further information

Mrs Reiss embarked on, and persisted with, the treatment planned with the psychologist. She was seen weekly for six weeks, then fortnightly for six sessions then at monthly intervals.

The emphasis remained on desensitization '*in vivo*'. For the first month Mrs Reiss co-operated well although her homework tended to be unsystematic. She kept her record of outgoings diligently but suddenly recorded higher anxiety ratings than previously.

Mrs Reiss' deterioration appeared to be due to her husband's responses to her treatment. On his return from the United States he tended to disparage her gains and on one occasion said that anyone ought to be able to do this without any help from the hospital. Mrs Reiss became extremely distressed about this and stopped practising. Several attempts to see Mr Reiss following this episode were unsuccessful. The next session was spend mainly in discussion of how she could deal with her husband's reaction and in devising ways in which praise from other family members could be maximized.

When the psychologist rang Mrs Reiss' home in order to change the next appointment Mr Reiss answered the telephone. He seemed more helpful than was the impression given by the patient. At one point he blamed himself for his wife's condition, stating that because of a heart attack and the medication he was prescribed, he was unable to give her 'enough love'. He said he often felt very depressed about himself. Mr Reiss was invited to attend the next session with his wife but he said that because of business pressures this would be unlikely.

For the next four weeks Mrs Reiss made considerable progress and was recording zero anxiety with 15 minute walks. She made two journeys on the underground and had used an escalator at a large shopping complex. However, over the following two weeks she again suffered a major setback, recording very high anxiety levels, stopping all practice and eventually retiring to her bed. During the next visit she complained that her husband distracted her when she was about to go out and gave her other jobs to do. The dose of propranolol had been increased by her general practitioner and she felt this was making her dizzy. She had recently spoken to someone who had 'blacked out' on similar medication to hers and was distressed by this. She gave the impression that when she was ill her husband became more considerate and behaved more 'benignly' to her.

Mrs Reiss then became very tearful and said that she knew what the 'real' problem was. It came as a complete surprise to the therapist when Mrs Reiss confessed that she was preoccupied with thoughts of her first husband and that she had never really overcome his death. She often visualized him in her imagination and 'spoke' to him when she was alone. Any mention of death or illness caused her to think immediately of him.

Much time in the next few sessions was spend in discussing her first husband's death and Mrs Reiss' feelings about him. Ways in which she might act more assertively with her present husband were also explored.

Mrs Reiss improved again and became more assertive with her husband. She complained that he was still not keen on her going out. The psychologist spoke on the telephone to Mr Reiss on one occasion and he was clearly angry with his wife. He accused her of not practising her 'homework' because she had a 'lazy nature' and stated that she was not ill. When the psychologist mentioned that Mrs Reiss had expressed some concern about his health (he also had gall bladder stones) he replied, 'It's my business if I die'. The psychologist responded sympathetically to Mr Reiss and urged him to encourage Mrs Reiss to go out.

Although Mrs Reiss' symptoms fluctuated, she is now improving steadily. At this stage it is useful to reconsider her case in order to see whether new lines of enquiry or treatment should be pursued.

Reformulation

Diagnosis

In addition to the agoraphobia, obesity, and hypertension it has become clear that Mrs Reiss has suffered from a longstanding, unresolved grief reaction following the death of her first husband. She has been unable to accept his death and has remained unusually preoccupied with his memory, which was immediately evoked by any reference to death or illness.

Aetiology

The problems that appeared to exist in Mr and Mrs Reiss' marriage have been confirmed by the contradictory reactions the psychologist observed when he spoke to Mr Reiss on the telephone. On one occasion he appeared sympathetic and expressed concern for his wife's illness and on another he blamed her completely for her problems. It is likely that Mr Reiss behaves in a way which tends to impede change in his wife. It would be shortsighted, however, to blame Mr Reiss' ambivalent attitude for the perpetuation of her symptoms. In a marital dyad a complex two-way pattern of interaction takes place with both partners contributing actively to the situation which exists at any one time. This state, although seeming unsatisfactory to an outsider, may represent a delicate balance which if disturbed could make matters worse, or at least the partners may fear they will become worse. In the case of Mrs Reiss one may hypothesize that her symptoms, by rooting her to her home, made it impossible for her to flee from her home and a relationship which was not satisfying her. Her symptoms seemed to embody her need to stay with the security she managed to create for herself after the war and a wish to escape from a troubled marriage. Mr Reiss is likely to have been aware of her dissatisfaction and his fear of being abandoned by her would make his behaviour directed towards discouraging change more understandable.

It has also been revealed that Mr Reiss has a serious heart condition which appears to have caused him considerable worry. Given Mrs Reiss' preoccupation with her first husband and her vulnerability to fear of death, this would have presumably been a considerable source of concern for her as well. It is surprising, in one so sensitive to illness, that she failed to mention her husband's heart condition about which he was obviously distressed. The reason for this omission is not clear, but perhaps it was due to an inability on her part to face the implications that he might die as well. Perhaps her unassertiveness with him was in part related to her fear that by resisting him she might hasten his demise.

Another factor which may have contributed to Mrs Reiss' illness is her daughter recently leaving her. Not only might this loss have been sad in itself, but also meant that she was left alone with her husband.

Further investigations

The importance of these, or other, aetiological and perpetuating factors should be explored by seeing the couple together, if this is possible.

Management

The psychiatrist should provide her with further opportunity to
mourn her first husband's death by focusing on issues which
evoke memories of him. It has also become increasingly clear
that Mrs Reiss should be seen with her husband and more pressure should be brought to bear on them to attend together.

Prognosis

Mrs Reiss should continue to improve. However, the scope for
improvement will depend upon the possibility of incorporating
her husband in the treatment. It seems unlikely that she will ever
completely come to terms with her losses, which have been so
numerous and profound.

Postscript

Although Mr Reiss never attended the out-patient department,
Mrs Reiss continued to make progress with her agoraphobic
symptoms despite some minor setbacks. She explored some of
the ways in which she contributed to her husband's irritability
with her. Thoughts about her first husband and her 'unforgiving
nature' were identified as probably having an influence. Soon
after, Mr Reiss expressed the desire to emigrate to Florida which
was contrary to Mrs Reiss' wishes. This had been a point of con-
tention for some time but not previously mentioned by the
patient. She responded to this more assertively than previously
but the question remained unresolved at the end of treatment.

Mrs Reiss was discharged from the clinic after nine months,
much improved. She was able to walk anywhere with marginal
anxiety and could drive to any point in Manchester. She was still
unable to approach escalators with total confidence but felt that
she could 'treat herself' for this. Her gains had been steady over
the previous three months. Thoughts of her first husband were
less frequent and she felt she had resolved much concerning his
loss.

Assessing the seriousness of a psychotic episode—the case of George Forrester, aged 51

Presenting complaint

Mrs Forrester telephoned the duty psychiatrist to ask for her husband to be seen urgently, because he had become increasingly depressed. When he attended his last out-patient appointment two weeks previously, his psychiatrist prescribed imipramine. In spite of taking this regularly his mood had deteriorated and on the previous day he had made a noose of his tie, pulled it tight around his neck and then released it. On the day of the telephone call, while Mrs Forrester was visiting her mother, he broke a neighbour's window, cutting his wrist. On her return home she found a suicide note he had written to their 10-year-old son. The duty psychiatrist confirmed that Mr Forrester had been a patient of the hospital for several years and advised Mrs Forrester to bring him directly to the out-patients' department. When they arrived, the following information was obtained from Mrs Forrester.

She had become increasingly worried about her husband and had therefore brought forward his out-patient appointment so that he was seen two weeks before. However, in spite of seeing his psychiatrist and being prescribed an antidepressant, his mood had deteriorated. He became increasingly taciturn and looked tense and miserable. He also began to talk more about how hopeless he felt about their marriage and began to sleep very badly. She had woken up on several occasions to find him sitting upright in bed during the early hours of the morning. At these times he stared bleakly out of the window. The previous week he woke up at 1 a.m. and said to her 'Oh Christ, I can't think why you married me'. His appetite diminished considerably and he left at least half of his meal untouched. In contrast to his increasing withdrawal and apathy, Mr Forrester had begun to make more frequent sexual advances towards her over the last two weeks.

Mrs Forrester did not bring the suicide note with her. She could not remember exactly what it contained but it was written to their son and was basically an apology for feeling so hopeless.

The psychiatrist was unable to read Mr Forrester's records in detail before he examined him. However, he managed to obtain the following information from the summaries of Mr Forrester's previous admissions to hospital.

Family history

His father was a general practitioner who died at the age of 59 from a coronary, when Mr Forrester was 12 years old. He was said to have suffered from 'neurasthenia' and he spent the last year of his life in a nursing home. Although he was a rather distant man, he occasionally showed a very violent temper and shouted at his family. Mr Forrester's mother died at the age of 79, when Mr Forrester was aged 49. She was described as a kind, loving housewife who was very patient with the whole family. He had three siblings. Avril was eight years older than Mr Forrester, unmarried, and died at the age of 36 from pneumonia. Alfred, who was six years older, was an airman who was shot down and missing, presumed dead, at the end of the Second World War when Mr Forrester was 17. There was also an unmarried brother, Jack, two years older than Mr Forrester. Jack had been admitted for a few months to a nursing home when he was 48 with a 'nervous breakdown'. Apart from occasionally appearing a little 'odd', he had no further relapses and continued to lead a full and independent life.

Personal history

Mr Forrester was born in Nottingham where he spent a rather isolated childhood. He received private tuition until he was eight years old, when he started to attend the local boarding school. He never made any close friends and immersed himself in his studies. He passed the entrance examination to Cambridge when he was 18 and read history. After he obtained his degree he taught history for a few years in a number of schools, but eventually decided to give this up. He then spent a few years travelling around South Africa before he returned to the United Kingdom, where he took a year's course in administration. For the past 15 years he had worked as a hospital archivist.

He met his wife, who was two years older than him, when he was 37. They married soon after meeting and their relationship was described as 'reasonably stable' until the last few years. They had one child, a son aged 10.

Past medical history

At the age of four he fractured his leg in a car accident and this resulted in a permanent limp.

Past psychiatric history

Mr Forrester had two brief spells of psychotherapy when he was aged 37 and 40. From the age of 42, he experienced fairly regular episodes of psychiatric illness, which required hospital in-patient treatment about every two years. On most of these admissions, he was diagnosed as suffering from depression, but on one occasion a diagnosis of schizophrenia was made, and on two further occasions mania had been diagnosed. Over the years he had received tricyclic antidepressants, haloperidol, electroconvulsive treatment and lithium carbonate. He had been maintained on lithium carbonate for the last two years and attended the out-patient department every few months in order to monitor both his mental state and his medication. Although his mood fluctuated during this time most of the comments written about him by the doctors who saw him referred to his 'rather strange personality'.

Previous personality

His wife described him as a withdrawn, shy, socially inept man who made few friends.

Mental state examination

Appearance and general behaviour

Mr Forrester was a tall, slightly stooped, gaunt-looking man with long, unkempt white hair. His shirt collar was undone and he was not wearing a tie but he was otherwise dressed tidily. He sat with his head in his hands and looked tense and extremely dejected. His face had an agonized expression on it and he frequently grimaced. He spent the whole interview sitting still, looking at the floor.

Talk

It was impossible to have a conversation with Mr Forrester. He answered most questions by shouting 'I don't know'. When he spoke more fluently it was at a normal rate. He appeared to have formal thought disorder: when he was talking about his thoughts he said 'I have no longer a mind of my own. I fear for the Queen's safety. I am not fit to be seen or heard'.

Mood

Mr Forrester looked and sounded extremely miserable, but when he was asked if he was feeling depressed he shook his head vigorously. However, when this question had been put to him several times he agreed that he had been depressed. He broke down and sobbed after he described what was happening to his thoughts.

Thought content

When he was asked how he felt he shouted 'I don't know'. He shook his head when he was asked whether he felt angry or frightened. He was then asked whether he felt aggressive towards anyone and he shouted 'Only with myself'. When the possibility of admission to hospital was suggested, he shouted out 'No, no, no!'.

Abnormal beliefs and interpretation of events

After the possibility of admission had been raised he went on to say 'I don't know who my father is. I don't know what to think of him. I don't know whether he is a monster, too'. The psychiatrist then asked him whether he thought that he was a monster and he replied 'Yes'. When he was asked what sort of a monster he said 'God alone knows. He ought to, he made me'.

When he was asked about his thoughts Mr Forrester said 'I think people can transfer their thoughts to my mind to make me do things I don't want to do, make me say things I don't want to say. I have no longer a mind of my own'.

Abnormal experiences

When he was talking about how he felt, Mr Forrester said 'I feel as if I'm being pulled apart by some kind of a force'. He was then asked what this force was and replied 'Ask my brother. I feel as if I'm being driven into the ground like a stake, but I don't know by whom'.

Cognitive state

This was not formally tested.

Appraisal of illness

Mr Forrester was unable to discuss what was happening to him, but expressed clearly the belief that he did not need to be in hospital.

Physical examination

This was not performed in the out-patient department, but it was noted that Mr Forrester's left arm was bandaged, apparently because of lacerations.

Summary

Mr Forrester's presentation is of a recent, severe alteration in mood and behaviour which has culminated in two episodes of self-harm, one of which was associated with him writing a suicide note. These changes have occurred in the context of a long-standing, cyclical illness which has required fairly regular admission to hospital. The formulation will therefore need to address the severity of Mr Forrester's current state, the need for hospital admission and if necessary the possibility of invoking the Mental Health Act in order to obtain formal admission.

Formulation

Diagnosis

It is almost certain that Mr Forrester has developed an acute psychotic illness. First, his records show that he has had fairly regular episodes of psychotic illness over the last 10 years. Secondly, his wife describes a deterioration in his mood and general behaviour over the last few months. She says that he has become increasingly withdrawn, has begun to express ideas of hopelessness, and that his sleep and appetite have become seriously disturbed. These abnormalities have culminated in his suicide attempt. Thirdly, his mental state is extremely disturbed. He looks unhappy, is unable to give a coherent explanation for his recent behaviour and what he does say suggests that he has experienced delusions and feels the victim of some kind of persecution. For example, when he describes himself as feeling 'pulled apart by some kind of force' and 'being driven into the ground like a stake'.

The nature of the psychotic illness is uncertain, because it has features consistent with both an affective disorder and a schizophrenic disorder. Both of these diagnoses have been made during previous episodes and the information obtained from the summaries is unsufficient to resolve this uncertainty. However, it is his mood that appears to have been most affected by his illness which suggests it is more likely to be an affective psychosis. This likelihood is reinforced by the description of recent changes in his sleep and eating and the fact that his illness appears to have had a fairly regular periodicity.

On the other hand, a diagnosis of schizophrenia has been made previously and persecutory ideas are prominent in this episode. An even more suspicious symptom is his description of thought insertion, which is said to be pathognomonic of a diagnosis of schizophrenia. However, this is not necessarily the case since Schneider's 'first rank symptoms' of schizophrenia can be found in cases of mania, particularly in the acute stages. Although Mr Forrester has shown no obvious manifestations of a manic illness during this episode, this diagnosis has been made in the past. Furthermore, his heightened sexual activity, which contrasts with his general sense of retardation, raises the possibility that he has an admixture of depressive and manic symptoms which often occurs in acute affective illnesses.

Aetiology

Mr Forrester appears to have a familial predisposition to psychiatric illness. His father suffered from what the family describes as 'neurasthenia' which may have led to him spending the last year of his life in a nursing home. His brother has also had a 'nervous breakdown' which also required treatment in a nursing home. In addition to the possibility that Mr Forrester might have inherited a predisposition to psychiatric illness, it may be that exposure to his father's unpredictable and volatile mood also influenced his personality development. His wife described Mr Forrester as generally an isolated and depressive person. Although she did not meet him before he suffered his first psychiatric episode, this tendency towards isolation appears to extend back into his early childhood. This raises the possibility that Mr Forrester has a schizoid personality, which would colour any psychiatric illness he might develop.

No obvious precipitants of this episode have been identified His illness has previously shown a periodicity of approximately two years which is additional support for some underlying biological vulnerability. There is also the possibility that Mr Forrester has not been taking his medication as prescribed and that this might have contributed to his relapse.

Further investigations

In order to clarify the diagnosis it is necessary to define more clearly Mr Forrester's current mental state. It is also important to obtain more details of his mental state during previous admissions. This should show the extent to which his abnormal beliefs and behaviour are consistent with an affective or a schizophrenic illness.

A full physical examination needs to be performed, particularly in view of his efforts at self-harm.

It might also prove useful to find out more about the details of both his brother's and his father's psychiatric episodes. If they also showed features of a psychotic disorder this would increase the likelihood of a constitutional vulnerability.

More information is also required about his personal and developmental history. In particular the quality of academic degree he obtained and his reasons for changing his job would provide a clearer picture of his personality and his capabilities before his first episode of psychiatric illness.

Further detail is also needed about the events in Mr Forrester's life during the time leading up to this episode. Given Mrs Forrester's comments about his personality it would not be surprising to find that their marriage had been under considerable strain. It may also be relevant that his first serious psychiatric episode occurred at the time his son was born.

Blood levels of both imipramine and lithium will need to be obtained. These may show the extent to which Mr Forrester has been co-operating with his medical treatment.

Management

There are important clinical indications for admitting Mr Forrester immediately. First, he is suffering from a serious exacerbation of a psychiatric illness which warrants urgent treatment. Secondly, treatment as an out-patient has already failed to prevent a considerable deterioration. Thirdly, there is evidence to suggest that he is a danger to himself. Within the last 24 hours there have been two episodes of self-harm and he has written a suicide note to his son. These factors suggest that he should be admitted to hospital urgently and that when this takes place he will have to be closely observed. Finally, he neither thinks he is ill nor believes he needs psychiatric treatment. Since he is not only seriously ill, but also a considerable danger to himself as a result of this, Mr Forrester should be admitted to a ward where special attention can be paid to his nursing care. In view of the presumptive diagnosis his medication should also be continued in the previously prescribed doses until blood levels have been obtained. Mr Forrester's reaction to admission suggests that this might require formal procedures under section of the Mental Health Act if all attempts to gain his co-operation fail.

Prognosis

Although Mr Forrester is seriously ill, it seems likely that he will recover from this episode as he has done previously. What is uncertain is how long this recovery will take, how complete it will be, and how vulnerable Mr Forrester will remain to further relapses. A clearer picture should emerge once more information has become available.

Brief formulation

Mr Forrester is a 51-year-old married, hospital archivist who presents with a several months' history of emotional withdrawal, miserable thoughts, altered sleep, and reduced appetite. In spite of being prescribed imipramine these symptoms have worsened and he has tried to harm himself on two occasions. On examination, he is miserable, his thinking is disordered, and he describes strange experiences and beliefs which have a persecutory nature. He is otherwise unable to express these recent changes. Over the last nine years he has been admitted to psychiatric hospitals at two yearly intervals when he has generally been diagnosed as suffering from an affective illness.

Diagnosis

The most likely diagnosis is an affective psychosis. He currently shows a change in his mood and has disturbed sleep and appetite. Furthermore, his previous psychotic episodes are consistent with this diagnosis. It is less likely that he is suffering from a schizophrenic illness, even though he describes symptoms of persecution and possibly of thought insertion.

Aetiology

Mr Forrester's family history suggests a constitutional vulnerability to psychiatric illness. His isolated upbringing may also have contributed to his generally withdrawn personality, which might be a further vulnerability factor. There is also the possibility that Mr Forrester has not been taking his prescribed medication in adequate doses.

Further investigations

More information is required about Mr Forrester's previous psychiatric episodes and the events leading up to this presentation. A fuller picture of his early development and of his marital relationship is necessary. Finally, blood levels of lithium and imipramine are required.

Management

He needs to be admitted urgently to a ward where he can be closely observed and special attention paid to his nursing care. If necessary this will have to be as a formal patient. Treatment with imipramine and lithium carbonate should be continued.

Prognosis

Mr Forrester should recover from this episode with adequate treatment, but he seems vulnerable to further relapses in the future.

Further information

When the duty psychiatrist made clear his intention to admit him urgently, Mr Forrester agreed to come into hospital voluntarily. Following admission, it was possible to examine his psychiatric records in more detail and to obtain further information from him and from his wife, which allowed more detailed and accurate personal and past psychiatric histories to be obtained.

Personal history

Mr Forrester's early recollections were fairly happy ones. However, he had no memory of playing with any of his siblings nor of having any close friends. It became clearer that his father's psychiatric illness had been incapacitating and it caused him to spend the last year of his life in a nursing home. However no further details about this or his brother's illness were obtained.

Mr Forrester had always immersed himself in his studies to the exclusion of any social life. This continued at Cambridge, where he obtained a second class history degree in his finals. When he left Cambridge, he applied for war service but was rejected because of his limp. He then taught history for a few years. Although he found this initially quite enjoyable, he had considerable difficulty maintaining discipline and it was for this reason that he gave up teaching. It was then that he decided to take up a course in administration which he completed before he travelled to South Africa. He said that this was because he felt unsettled in England and when he left he had intended to settle in South Africa permanently. He found life there more relaxed and he was able to make several friends, but in spite of this he found himself missing England increasingly and he therefore returned after seven years. He remained unemployed for two years after he returned and then obtained his current job as a hospital archivist. He generally enjoyed his work, although he occasionally felt that he was 'stuck in a rut'. His employers described him as having been a 'painstaking and conscientious worker' and said that they never found any cause for concern about him until the time of his first 'breakdown' when they noticed an increasing number of errors in his work. At that time they also noticed him becoming quite withdrawn and on occasions either falling asleep or just wandering away from work. After his first admission to hospital he returned to work although there were several periods of sick leave during subsequent relapses. His employers were very sympathetic to his difficulties and kept his job open for him. However, he was transferred to another department for what were described as 'administrative reasons'. One advantage of his current job was that it provided Mr Forrester with a considerable amount of spare time to pursue his hobbies of writing short plays and poetry.

Before he met his wife he had several girlfriends, but none of these relationships were serious or intimate. His wife said that when she first met him she 'felt sorry for him', but also went on to say that she did not realize 'how difficult he could be' until after they married. She was particularly bothered by his tendency to withdraw from any active involvement in the family. Although they never had a frequent sexual relationship, this had become totally non-existent over the previous three years. Neither Mr nor Mrs Forrester expressed any concern about this aspect of their relationship.

When they married they had not planned to have any children

but Mr Forrester said that although he was not closely involved in his son's upbringing, he 'accepted' him and 'felt responsible' for him.

In addition to writing, his interests were intellectual and unusual. He had always been fascinated by languages and ,once began to learn Esperanto, out of which he developed ideas to create a language of his own. At the time of his first psychiatric breakdown he became interested in a religious cult that was attempting to reconcile all religions under one banner.

Past psychiatric history

Mr Forrester's first admission to a psychiatric hospital took place when he was 42. He was diagnosed as suffering from endogenous depression and was reported to have responded well to electro-convulsive treatment. A few months later, he was readmitted to another psychiatric hospital where a diagnosis of schizophrenia was made, based upon the presence of 'bizarre, delusional ideas'. However, it was noted at that time that these occurred in the context of a depressive mood. The diagnosis was subsequently changed to one of endogenous depression and he was given a further course of electro-convulsive therapy in addition to tri-fluoperazine and dothiepin. One year later, he was readmitted with a diagnosis of depression, which again responded to a course of electro-convulsive therapy. Two years later, he took an overdose of antidepressants and was readmitted to hospital.

Following this overdose he suffered a *grand mal* seizure. He later developed an elated mood with considerable activity, as a result of which a diagnosis of mania was made. At this time he was treated with haloperidol and he appeared to remain well for a further two years. He was then readmitted compulsorily for a four day period of assessment, which was extended to a one year treatment order on account of his continuing unpredictable behaviour. There were frequent comments in the notes about his becoming embroiled in arguments with staff over whether he needed to be in hospital or receive treatment. He was reported to have left the ward without warning on several occasions and the nursing staff found him very unco-operative. There were frequent comments in their records about their difficulty in getting to know him. The final diagnosis on this admission was mania.

Since his last admission Mr Forrester had often failed to keep his out-patient appointments and frequently wrote letters to the doctors who looked after him. These discussed, amongst other things, the value (or lack of it) that he placed upon his contact with the hospital, the psychological basis of illness, and other philosophical issues. His letter-writing appeared to alter during his 'manic' phase. The letters became not only more frequent and longer, but more rambling with some flight of ideas. For example, one letter described a profound religious experience, then personal and sexual experiences, then problems with medication, then a review of important biographical dates in his life and then a train journey. This was closely-written on five sides of paper in two colours of ink.

Further enquiry about the event leading up to Mr Forrester's recent deterioration revealed that he had started a refresher course on administration six months beforehand. However, he felt unable to continue after two days and gave it up. Mrs Forrester believed that his mood began to detiorate at about this time. No other specific stresses were revealed.

The various doctors who saw Mr Forrester and his wife in the out-patient department commented on Mrs Forrester's anxiety about her husband, in particular, the fact that she frequently telephoned the hospital to voice her worries about him. There were also comments about how his mood had fluctuated during the previous two years. However, most of their notes referred to his 'rather strange, withdrawn personality'.

Physical examination

A complete physical examination revealed evidence of weight loss, a superficial three-inch (7 cm) laceraton of his left arm, and a fixed flexion deformity of his right knee, but no other abnormality.

Special investigations

Mr Forrester's serum lithium level was 0.5 mmol/l. Although this was just within the therapeutic range for the laboratory (0.5–1.5 mmol/l) it was lower than the level Mr Forrester had maintained during the previous four years (0.6–0.8 mmol/l). His imipramine level was 43 mg/l and his desipramine level was 41 mg/l. (The combined total, 84 mg/l was sub-therapeutic for the laboratory: 150–300 mg/l.)

All other investigations were normal.

Mental state examination

Appearance and behaviour

Following his admission Mr Forrester took very little care of his appearance, and remained unkempt and unshaven. He ate poorly, which he attributed to an aversion to meat. He was reported to be sleeping restlessly. He developed no rapport with anyone on the ward and when interviewed he either paced restlessly around or sat upright, unblinking in a chair, staring at the floor with his legs crossed and hands clasped tensely.

Talk

During the first week, he offered no spontaneous conversation and always gave terse answers to questions. However, he became a little more forthcoming towards the end of his second week in hospital.

Mood

During the first week of his admission he consistently conveyed to the ward staff a sense of depressive desolation and hopelessness. He said that he felt as if he were in 'cold storage' and that admission to hospital had been 'an ordeal I have to experience' and although 'it could conceivably have a useful purpose in the long run', he saw his 'previous life as having been a preparation for this'. He thought that he deserved to have this experience and saw it as a punishment for having been rude to his father, as well as for having blasphemed when he was admitted to hospital four years previously. He made numerous allusions to suicide, saying that life was not worth living and that he would 'welcome the opportunity for suicide' because he would be 'better off out of the way'. One way of achieving this would be to 'sacrifice myself as a hero rather than being a coward' and he was therefore prepared to offer himself for 'euthanasia'.

Thought content

He expressed an interest in symbolism, which he thought conveyed messages. He gave as an example, 'a frog, which is ignorant of the underworld'. When asked to explain what this meant, he replied, 'it has something to do with croaking. If you croak you are finished'. He then said that he was reminded of this by someone who wore clothes with a picture of a frog on the back of them when he had attended a religious festival a few weeks previously.

Abnormal beliefs and interpretations of events

Mr Forrester seemed very suspicious and expressed the belief that he was being 'organized by someone else, possibly for historical purpose'. There seemed to him to be 'a purpose behind what was going on', although he did not know what this was and thought that 'only God could provide an answer'. He wondered if God had made use of the Devil to test him. A week after his admission, he said that at the time of his admission he 'felt framed' and 'imagined' that his room had been bugged. At that time he said that someone was listening because 'I gave a transmission, a couple of sonnets and a short poem in Russian. I wasn't going to give away any secrets—I can't remember what they were. It always comes back to loyalty'. He also said that he imagined he was the 'pretender to the throne'. In addition to these thoughts, he felt that everything had a double meaning 'like being in a film', but he was unable to elaborate any further on this. When efforts were made to establish how firmly he held these ideas, he always deflected this line of enquiry by saying that he used to believe these things or that they were imaginary.

Abnormal experiences

None were elicited.

Cognitive state

This was never formally tested apart from confirming that Mr Forrester was orientated in time and space.

Appraisal of illness

Soon after his admission Mr Forrester said 'I don't honestly feel unwell'. Ten days later, he said 'I was certainly ill one week ago, but I am sane now'.

Nursing observations

All the nursing staff commented on his rather cold, empty, and distant personality which made it difficult for them to empathize with his situation.

Although not all the questions raised in the intial formulation have been answered a consistent view of Mr Forrester extending back over nearly 10 years, has emerged. The reader should now be able to put this together. It might be particularly interesting to consider the outcome and to compare this with the following prognosis and the postscript.

Reformulation

Diagnosis

There is now little doubt that Mr Forrester is suffering from an affective psychosis. He conveys an intensity of hopelessness about himself and his future and the many delusions he describes all have a distinctive depressive colouring and appear to have arisen out of this mood change, rather than being the cause of it. These delusions are quite persecutory, since he believes he is at the centre of some religious conspiracy and that he is being 'organized' by some outside agent. In addition they have a grandiose quality because Mr Forrester believes he has been singled out and is going to be a part of history.

This grandiose quality raises the suspicion that there is a manic element to Mr Forrester's current illness. This is reinforced by another symptom suggestive of mania that has been noted. Mr Forrester makes an association between a frog, the underworld and death in a characteristic 'flight of ideas' linked by, amongst other things, the pun on the word 'croaked'. This admixture of manic and depressive symptoms, in the context of a chronic episodic illness with both depressive and manic swings, defines the affective disturbance as 'mixed type'.

It seems that Mr Forrester may have experienced 'thought broadcasting' early on during his admission. Although this is one of the 'first rank symptoms' of schizophrenia, as has been discussed before, such symptoms can occur during a manic illness. This explanation is further supported by the previous descriptions of 'bizarre' thoughts which have occurred in earlier episodes, which have nevertheless followed the pattern of a cyclical affective illness.

The additional information that has been obtained also suggests that Mr Forrester has a schizoid personality. He appears to have had a life-long tendency of social withdrawal and isolation and has never had any intense emotional involvement with another person, including his wife and son. In particular he described his relationship with his son in terms of responsibility, rather than concern. Furthermore, he has always shown interest in rather abstruse matters, such as developing a new language or the philosophical aspects of religion. Although these features are not in themselves necessarily manifestations of a psychiatric disturbance, when they play such a prominent part in an individual's character they suggest considerable eccentricity. These schizoid attributes seem to have coloured Mr Forrester's psychotic episodes when they have occurred, giving them what has been referred to as their 'bizarre' or 'schizophrenic' qualities.

Aetiology

The importance of a familial factor in Mr Forrester's illness, is reinforced by establishing the severity of his father's illness. He may also have inherited a schizoid tendency from his father which could well have been reinforced by his rather isolated upbringing.

Mr Forrester's recent deterioration appears to have been associated with his starting a course which he failed to complete. From his wife's account, it is possible that this set-back triggered off this episode, although it could also have been an early symptom of it.

There is also the likelihood that Mr and Mrs Forrester's marriage is under considerable stress as a result of his personality and his vulnerability to illness. She has made several criticisms about his lack of involvement and has expressed disappointment at the way their marriage has turned out. Although no specific details have been revealed, it is also possible that Mrs Forrester has been putting her husband under increasing pressure on account of this. Given his personality he would find it very difficult to cope with intense emotional demands and this might have also been a factor contributing to his deterioration.

His previous records contain no mention of any specific environmental triggers. However, his first psychotic episode did occur within the first year of his son's birth and it is a reasonable speculation that the additional emotional pressures of a small child might also have contributed to this episode.

Finally, the blood tests have shown that his medication is at the lower therapeutic level. Given the stresses discussed above and his apparent cyclical vulnerability, this relative lack of medication may also have contributed to his relapse.

Further investigations

It will be important to obtain a much more detailed account of Mr and Mrs Forrester's relationship. This should include an estimation of its strengths as well as its weaknesses. It is unclear how much support Mrs Forrester is giving her husband and whether she may be making unrealistic demands of him, given his personality and psychological vulnerability.

More details should be obtained about the course which appears to have been associated with Mr Forrester's deterioration. In particular, it should be clarified whether this did in fact precede his relapse.

Management

Mr Forrester will need to remain in a ward where he can be given high intensity nursing care until he is no longer a danger to himself and shows a capacity to co-operate with treatment. It would probably be wise to keep him there until it is clear that he is not developing a full-blown manic episode, particularly in the light of his previous difficulty in co-operating with treatment.

The possibility of electro-convulsive treatment should be considered, since it has been shown to be useful for Mr Forrester in the past. However, he has already shown signs of improvement during his first two weeks in hospital, when he was known to be receiving adequate doses of imipramine and lithium carbonate. Although a case can be put forward for giving electro-convulsive treatment as well, there seems little point in doing this while he continues to improve. He will need to continue with imipramine for at least nine months after he has recovered from this episode and to continue with his lithium carbonate indefinitely, because he has shown vulnerability to regular, serious relapses. This will require close monitoring to maintain it within what has been shown to be the therapeutic range for Mr Forrester.

Mr Forrester should be encouraged to return to work following recovery. Assuming that his employers are prepared to keep his job available for him, his work environment seems particularly suitable for someone of his personality and vulnerability in that it appears to be emotionally undemanding.

Further treatment of the couple will probably need to be educational, helping them to avoid situations which might precipitate further breakdown. The need for this has already been demonstrated by the frequency with which Mrs Forrester telephones the hospital to communicate her anxiety about her husband. It may be that more fundamental interpersonal issues will become aired, but this could have disastrous consequences given Mr Forrester's personality and it may be better to avoid too deep an exploration.

It may be necessary to advise Mr Forrester to avoid certain situations to which he is vulnerable. An example of this might turn out to be courses like the one that was associated with his current deterioration.

Prognosis

It is likely that Mr Forrester will recover from this episode after a few months in hospital as he has done on previous occasions. However, there is a considerable risk that he will swing into a manic phase once his depression lifts. If this follows the previous pattern, then it will be associated with considerable conflict between Mr Forrester and the ward staff. In the longer term Mr Forrester appers to be vulnerable to a relapse at intervals of approximately two years. The possibility of preventing this will depend upon very close monitoring of both his mental state, potential social triggers and medication.

Given his employer's previous co-operation and the lack of

stress placed upon him at work, it is likely that Mr Forrester will be able to return there.

There is a clear danger that Mr and Mrs Forrester's marriage will break down, partly on account of his illness and partly because of his personality difficulties. The likelihood of this happening cannot be ascertained until more information has been obtained about the couple's relationship.

Postscript

Mr Forrester remained in hospital for five months and his recovery was a stormy one. He had marked mood swings, which might have been partly attributable to a muddle over his medication. He embarked upon a relationship with a female patient which caused considerable distres for his wife. However, his mental state was controlled with a mixture of lithium carbonate, imipramine and chlorpromazine. In spite of improvement, he remained an extremely impenetrable individual, who continued to be preoccupied with philosophical conundrums.

Efforts were made to embark upon conjoint assessment and counselling, but these were not maintained. Mrs Forrester had considerable difficulty in attending, which was heightened by her husband's flirtation on the ward. Eventually Mr Forrester went on a fortnight's holiday with his wife and returned to his home and to work without reporting back to the ward.

Six years later Mr Forrester had not required readmission. He suffered several relapses during which he again wrote detailed and involved letters to his psychiatrist, but these were controlled by an increase in his medication. He managed to cope with the stresses imposed by his mother-in-law's death and his retirement. According to his employers, he continued to function well until his retirement, when he was offered part-time, unpaid employment.

On two occasions, Mrs Forrester 'offered' to leave her husband because she believed that she 'contributed to his illness'. However, over several years their relationship appeared to settle down considerably.

Following Mr Forrester's discharge his psychiatrist received a letter from Mr Forrester's brother, Jack, which suggested that Mr Forrester's problem was due to 'a mixture of drug intoxication and vitamin imbalance'. Jack also suggested that this had probably contributed to their father's illness. This letter was as disjointed and obscure as Mr Forrester's had been during his manic phase.

10

Relapse of psychosis—the case of Mr Butler, aged 32

Presenting complaint

Mr Butler was referred to a psychiatric emergency clinic by his general practitioner because he was 'going through another episode of suicidal thoughts'. The general practitioner stated that for about five years he had suffered from 'profound mental disturbance', with withdrawal, depersonalization, depression, and paranoia'. A confident diagnosis of paranoid schizophrenia was made in the emergency clinic, the risk of suicide was noted, and Mr Butler was referred to see a consultant in the out-patient department. The consultant thought that the correct diagnosis was depressive illness in a sensitive personality and made arrangements for admission.

Mr Butler himself had the following complaints—that his house was being bugged, that electronic noises were being made, and that wind effects were occurring outside the house when there was no wind. He also said that he had been frightened when 'something happened in my head like a shock wave'. The police were somehow mixed up with it, he thought. The history, obtained during the course of a two month admission, was as follows.

Mr Butler had been becoming hard of hearing for about 10 years. Five years before admission he became preoccupied with the idea that people were staring at him and that the police were following him. His beer drinking increased and, later that year, he was arrested by the police for being drunk and disorderly which convinced him that his suspicions of the police were correct.

Four years before admission Mr Butler took an overdose of a prescribed hypnotic whilst feeling 'depressed', and was admitted to a psychiatric hospital for the first time. He did not return to his job and was readmitted after three months. Mr Butler had then worked only intermittently in a succession of jobs, each shorter than the last. He was again arrested by the police on a drunk and disorderly charge and shortly after this, 18 months before the present admission, his feeling that the police were everywhere, putting 'pressure' on him had become so intense that he felt that he could not work.

Eight months before admission he cut his wrists with a razor blade and then made preparations to hang himself, although eventually deciding against doing so. He was again admitted to a psychiatric hospital, via a casualty department, but discharged himself after three days.

Since that time he had not worked but occupied himself at home reading magazines and doing crossword puzzles. He described himself as feeling continually worried and depressed.

Family history

Mr Butler's father, aged 63, had recently retired on medical grounds from the post office where he was a sorting office supervisor, but continued working as a part-time clerk in a builder's yard. He suffered from hypertension and angina. Mr Butler described his father as being a self-contained rather quiet man. He was in the habit of going to the pub twice a week with his son, and they shared an interest in football. Mr Butler's mother was also 63. She seemed a more outgoing woman who was the 'boss' of the family and 'doted' on Mr Butler. She had continued to work part-time as a school dinner-lady after she passed the age of retirement. Mr Butler had two siblings. (A first-born child, a brother, had died at birth). An older brother, married with six children, had emigrated to Australia, where he was working as a storeman. An older sister was married to a local electrician and had one child.

Mr Butler described his upbringing as having been 'warm and happy'. There was no family history of psychiatric disorder but a cousin had epilepsy and was described as being 'violent'.

Personal history

Mr Butler had lived throughout his life in a market town in the north of England. He was born in hospital by Caesarean section after a trial of labour had failed because of pelvic disproportion. There were no other perinatal complications. He was an unusually shy and timid child who became anxious easily. He disliked being alone but otherwise his development was normal, he enjoyed the company of other children, and particularly liked sports. After some initial apprehension he enjoyed school and was always a model pupil. He got on with everyone, both teachers and pupils, and became a prefect at secondary school. His academic record was good and he passed three O levels in history, art, and technical drawing at the age of 16. He wanted to stay on at school but his mother insisted that he went out to work in order to supplement the family income.

Mr Butler joined an off-licence chain after leaving school at the age of 16, and worked in the stock-taking department for 12 years. His work entailed travelling and making a complete on-the-spot inventory of the stock of individual shops, estimating its value. His ability to perform rapid calculations, his reliability, and, especially, his probity were much thought off and he was promoted to a position of seniority, shortly before his first breakdown.

There was an occasion when Mr Butler was 11, when he had engaged in mutual masturbation with another boy at school. At the age of 14 he experienced his first ejaculation. He was however very shy with girls and despite occasional 'dates' did not even kiss a girl until he was 20 years old. When he was aged 16 Mr Butler became infatuated with a young woman who lived locally and he would stand outside her house to try and catch glimpses of her undressing. On several occasions he stood deliberately close behind her at the bus stop and rubbed his body against hers. For a few years after this he would rub himself against, or touch knees with, women who attracted him when he was travelling on crowded trains. This activity did not outlast his adolescence and it never led to police attention. In his early twenties Mr Butler did, however, exhibit himself on one occasion, after drinking heavily.

Mr Butler had one experience of sexual intercourse, with his only girlfriend at the age of 22. They split up shortly afterwards. At the time of admission his only sexual outlet was masturbation. He masturbated two to three times a week usually whilst looking at 'girlie' magazines. He kept a collection of these and felt humiliated when, shortly before admission, his father discovered them.

Mr Butler had been a regular beer drinker, like his father since adolescence. His occupation encouraged his drinking but it was only towards the end of his work for the off-licence chain that he began to drink heavily every day, both at lunch-time and in the evening. Mr Butler did not have enough money to drink every day for some time before his admission, but developed the habit of drinking five pints of beer or more every Saturday and Sunday.

Life situation

Mr Butler and his parents had lived throughout his life in a three bedroomed council flat. He contributed some rent, but did very little at home, relying on his mother to clean his room, the cooking, and the washing.

Past medical history

Deafness was first noticed more than 10 years before.

Past psychiatric history

Mr Butler first saw a psychiatrist at the age of 28 when he was admitted as a day patient following medical treatment for an overdose of barbiturate. He attended hospital daily for three weeks and a diagnosis of 'acute paranoid reaction in a sensitive schizoid personality' was made. He was given no medication. Alcohol was thought to be a precipitant and he was advised to reduce his drinking. He was referred to an out-patient therapy group.

Informal in-patient admission 'for investigations' was arranged three months later. Mr Butler was in hospital for three weeks and on one occasion during this admission he was interviewed under the influence of methadrine. He was given no regular medication and the notes stated that there was 'no overt evidence of paranoid psychosis manifested on the ward' and 'no evidence of alcoholism'. Out-patient follow-up was recommended, but Mr Butler did not attend.

The third previous admission followed medical treatment for self-inflicted wrist lacerations, as already described. Mr Butler discharged himself after five days during which he received no drug treatment. The diagnosis of 'reactive depression related to feelings of sexual inadequacy' was made.

Previous personality

His mother described him as having always been 'very shy and sensitive. An introvert'. However, he was held in high esteem at work and school, and 'never lost a day's work'. She remarked also on his obedience, his many male friends, and his lack of girl-friends. Mr Butler preferred to stay at home when he could and once described himself as 'a bird who can't leave the nest'.

Mental state examination

Appearance and general behaviour

Mr Butler was a short, nice looking man of athletic build. His clothes were clean and his hair short and neatly combed. He sat in a tense posture and moved his body very little, although he smiled a lot. His voice was soft, and rather slow. He was rather passive during the interview, but ready to do anything that was asked of him.

Talk

His talk was normal, if slightly monosyllabic.

Mood

Mr Butler seemed slightly tense but was not overtly agitated. He described himself as 'a bit on the low side'. His appetite was normal and his weight steady. He had difficulty in falling asleep and his ruminations (to be described below) were worse at night. He woke late rather than earlier, and he had no diurnal variation of mood. His suicide preoccupations had disappeared after admission.

Thought content

Mr Butler's conversation constantly reverted to the police who he thought were watching and following him. In situations where he felt less guarded Mr Butler would explain that the police were interested in his sexual activities either because they knew of his previous frotteurism or because he was considered to be homosexual or, sometimes, because 'they think I will assault a child'.

These thoughts were so persistent that they interfered with Mr Butler's attention.

Abnormal beliefs and interpretation of events

Mr Butler imbued many aspects of his environment with abnormal significance feeling it to be filled with personal references to himself. When he saw a child he thought that the police had arranged for the child to be there as a test of his sexuality. He also thought that the television and the newspapers made disguised reference to his predicament, for example by broadcasting songs in which the word 'baby' was used.

Mr Butler believed that he could tell that his case was well-known to a person by the way that person looked at him, or by the way that fellow patients held the trays at dinner, or by gestures that they made with their hands. Casual conversations that he overheard took on a special meaning for him, and indeed such a conversation had precipitated his recent overdose.

He was convinced that his parents' flat was bugged, and that he was being observed by television cameras controlled by the police.

Mr Butler had, in fact, recently imagined having sex with children but believed that the police had put these thoughts into his mind. He had also occasionally linked the exacerbation of his ruminations at night with the upstairs neighbour turning off the lights, and said, once, that this man could 'turn the switch on me'.

Abnormal experiences

One of Mr Butler's complaints, as already mentioned, was of visual 'wind effects' in the absence of wind. These only lasted a day and were closely associated with hearing noises in his ears like 'wind or electronic noise'. These noises never sounded like words but were usually described as 'ringing' and felt by Mr Butler to originate in his ears.

Cognitive state

Mr Butler's orientation, attention, and recall were normal. His retention of a short address was poor. Serial subtraction was performed by him accurately and unusually quickly. He seemed of above average intelligence.

Appraisal of illness

Mr Butler was curiously ambivalent about the nature of his condition. Whilst being convinced that his suspicions of the police were well-founded, he would, at the same time, say that they were too fantastic to be true and that he had a 'complex'.

Physical examination

The only abnormalities detected were short sight, fully corrected by spectacles, and bilateral deafness, worse on the left. Sound was conducted better through bone than air in both ears.

Summary

Mr Butler is a 32-year-old single, unemployed man who lives with his parents in a small council flat. He has a 10-year-old history of increasing deafness, and a five-year history of fluctuating ideas of references and persecutory beliefs, especially involving the police. He has made two recent attempts on his life, and is a heavy drinker. As a result of his disturbance he has had multiple admissions which have resulted in a variety of diagnoses and have not led to effective treatment. The first priority for the admitting doctor is to formulate the diagnosis and this will entail correctly clarifying the signs and symptoms of Mr Butler's disorder.

Formulation

Diagnosis

Mr Butler has delusions of reference. He is also possibly hallucinated: he has described inexplicable visual experiences (seeing plants moving outside the window when there was no wind) and hearing 'electronic noises'. The noises which he locates in his ear may be related to his deafness, and be due to a dysfunction of his ear. However tinnitus is unlikely to occur in conductive deafness, and these may be auditory hallucinations.

The prominence of delusions in Mr Butler's illness, coupled with the absence of other disabling signs and symptoms of psychosis, justify the descriptive term paranoid state or paranoid psychosis. (Both usages of the term—the original one of 'delusional', and the more modern one of relating to ideas of persecution—are applicable to Mr Butler.)

Paranoid states may occur alone or in combination with the signs and symptoms of some organic psychoses, depression or of schizophrenia.

There is no evidence that Mr Butler has ever suffered from epilepsy, or that he has ever abused drugs (two common causes of an organic paranoid state) nor is there any sign of cognitive impairment. There is therefore no support for the diagnosis of organic psychosis.

Although it is uncommon for a depressive psychosis to take this form, this does sometimes happen in patients with sensitive or suspicious pre-morbid personality traits. Where the pre-morbid personality is markedly abnormal even quite mild depression may produce a paranoid state.

A depressive psychosis is consistent with Mr Butler's complaints of feeling depressed and his ruminations about previous minor sexual transgressions. However, Mr Butler's suicide attempts are not diagnostically specific as despair about the future may also occur in sufferers from other serious psychiatric disorders, such as schizophrenia, and there is little other evidence of primary depression. Mr Butler has not lost weight, he has had no diurnal variation of mood and no sleep disturbance. He did not feel he was to blame about his previous sexual behaviour, but felt that he was the object of unfair discrimination by the police on account of it.

Persecutory beliefs which arise in sensitive individuals like Mr Butler but are due to depression, usually disappear when the depression lifts. Mr Butler's mood, however, appears to have lightened quite quickly after hospital admission without a corresponding change in his delusions. A depressive disorder is not therefore a likely cause of his symptoms.

None of Mr Butler's symptoms are inconsistent with schizophrenia (it would be the paranoid sub-type that was applicable in this case), but there is no definite evidence of this disorder. Although some of Mr Butler's delusions (such as his conviction that patients know about his previous sex offences) are 'primary' in that they were not prompted by abnormal experiences, it is not clear whether his first delusion (that the police were following him) was based on a misperception or whether it was a delusional inference from a normal perception. The latter, a 'delusional perception', is characteristic of schizophrenia, but the former is not.

On one occasion, Mr Butler said 'The police put these thoughts (sexual thoughts towards children) in my head'. This was taken by the experienced examining psychiatrist to be a report of thought insertion, which, since it is one of Schneider's first-rank symptoms, would confirm the diagnosis of schizophrenia if present. However, without knowing how the thoughts were put into Mr Butler's head it is possible that he simply meant that some things that the police did suggested these thoughts to him.

A paranoid state characterized by delusions but not hallucinations ('paranoia') may sometimes result from the insidious elaboration of normal preoccupations until these dominate the patient's thinking and give rise to delusional beliefs about, and misinterpretations of, the patient's experience. The development of Mr Butler's suspicions about the police have this character. They developed in the context of his exaggerated guilty ruminations about past sexual deviations, and were exacerbated by his arrest on a charge of being drunk and disorderly. Chance sightings of policemen were subsequently explained by this belief: they were on the look-out for him, and knew his movements because they had installed bugging devices in his flat. The police's interest in him was also used to explain difficulties in relationships with workmates (who were 'in the know').

However, it is usual for paranoia to be based on a series of deductions, which appear plausible on first acquaintance. The beliefs are often, for this reason, in areas which are particularly open to doubt such as religion, physical health, or justice. Mr Butler gives several instances of new extensions of this delusional system that are arrived at as sudden convictions without any proper evidence—for example, that the way a fellow patient held his tray *showed* that he was 'in the know'.

To summarize, there are points against all possible types of paranoid states, except paranoid schizophrenia. However, apart from possible thought insertion, there are no definite pathognomic features of schizophrenia and the diagnosis must therefore be said to be tentative. This is not an unusual situation since many of these features, such as thought disorder and social deterioration, are less marked in the paranoid than the other subtypes of schizophrenia.

Aetiology

These can only be determined when a definite diagnosis has been made but there are some of obvious potential importance.

Mr Butler has been a heavy weekend beer drinker for a number of years, and increased his consumption as his illness deteriorated although apparently in response to his symptoms rather than as a cause of them. There was no evidence that he was physically dependent on alcohol. However, regular heavy drinking is known to contribute to the development of paranoid states.

Mr Butler was timid and unusually prone to anxiety as a child. In adolescence he was abnormally shy and unassertive. These are some of the features of a schizoid personality. The latter predisposes to the development of schizophrenia. His lack of social experience, limited social contact and sexual naïveté are likely, anyway, to have facilitated the development of his eccentric ideas and increased his anxiety in social encounters. Mr Butler's deafness may also have increased his social anxiety and provided opportunities for misinterpretation of other people's remarks.

There is no family history of schizophrenia and the abuse of drugs can also be ruled out of the possible causes. However, Mr Butler did have a complicated birth and perinatal trauma is probably a vulnerability factor.

The factors considered may all have contributed to Mr Butler first becoming ill, although none account for the timing of its onset. The likely precipitants are all psychological and include the psychological stress of changing his job to one involving more responsibility.

A separate consideration, more important for practical management, is what causes Mr Butler's relapses. Are there precipitants of relapse suggested by Mr Butlers' history? Current stresses at home, drinking, difficulties at work and concern about sexuality should all be considered. The history of the present illness obtained so far is not sufficiently clear for any of these factors to be singled out.

The content of Mr Butler's delusions is strongly influenced by his concern about his sexuality but it cannot be concluded from this that Mr Butler's conflict about his sexual feelings is an especially important source of stress.

Further investigations

Mr Butler's deafness needs assessment with a view to treatment. In practice it is probably best that he is referred to an ear, nose, and throat surgeon for this.

Several areas of the history need further investigation. Knowledge of Mr Butler's development and pre-morbid activities and interests is somewhat sketchy, and a confident diagnosis about his pre-morbid personality cannot be made. Nor is the history of the illness sufficiently well documented for the aetiologically important factors to be made out. It would also be useful to interview Mr Butler together with his family in order to form some impression of how they interact, and ascertain whether stress at home may have contributed to his illness.

Some features of Mr Butler's mental state, particularly the nature of his abnormal experiences, need clarification. For example, is he auditorily hallucinated?

Another important investigation is to observe Mr Butler's response to treatment, including hospital admission. The effects of living away from home, of increased social contact, of reducing alcohol consumption, and of improved auditory acuity (assuming that it is treatable) also need to be tested.

Blood should be sent as a routine for syphilis serology, and urine for a drug screen. A routine physical examination should be carried out to exclude the possibility of concurrent physical illness.

Management

Mr Butler's management will depend on a more precise determination of diagnosis and aetiology.

In the short term, a decision has already been made to admit him partly because of his suicidal preoccupations. Although these have disappeared since admission it is wise not to forget them until Mr Butler has been effectively treated. Medical and nursing staff should therefore be particularly alert to any deterioration in Mr Butler's mood. Medication may be started once a definite view has been formed about diagnosis. It is important too, that Mr Butler does not become more disabled as a result of inactivity on the ward. An occupational therapy programme may help to prevent this, especially if in the longer term occupation is available relevant to his work.

Making available other social roles, such as patients' representative or work co-ordinator plus everyday activities, such as cooking or laundering, may also reduce 'desocialization'.

Prognosis

This cannot be determined accurately until a definite diagnosis is made and appropriate treatment begun. However, it can be said that, as Mr Butler recovered from two previous episodes, the prognosis for this episode is good but the likelihood of recurrence is high. Mr Butler's deteriorating work history also suggests that despite symptomatic recovery, he may be becoming socially disabled.

Brief formulation

Mr Butler is a 32-year-old unemployed Englishman who has a 10-year old history of increasing deafness and a five-year history of deterioration in his work ability. He has had three episodes of suspiciousness and persecutory beliefs with occasional, less clear-cut abnormal experiences. There is suggestive evidence that he had a schizoid personality pre-morbidly.

Diagnosis

The most likely diagnosis is paranoid schizophrenia, but an atypical depressive illness coloured by his schizoid personality is also a possibility.

Aetiology

His pre-morbid personality probably also predisposed him to the illness, as probably did his deafness. Heavy drinking and concern about his own sexuality may also have contributed. It is less clear what has triggered subsequent episodes. There is no family history of schizophrenia.

Further investigations

Investigation of his deafness, and further clarification of the history of Mr Butler's mental state are required. Routine screening investigations should also be carried out.

Management

Whilst investigations are proceeding in hospital, Mr Butler's mood should be regularly assessed in view of his previous thoughts of suicide. Regular daily activities, relevant to Mr Butler's daily life, should be made available with the expectation that Mr Butler should become engaged in them to prevent de-socialization. Appropriate medication should be started once a definite diagnosis is made.

Prognosis

The prognosis for recovery from this episode is good, but relapse is likely in the long term.

Further information

Mr Butler's parents saw the doctor on one occasion but they were reluctant to be involved in further interviews which seemed to them to be critically scrutinizing either their past or present family relationships.

More detailed historical information came to light in subsequent interviws with Mr Butler, however, and of course the results of treatment and the effects of the passage of time also became apparent. Mr Butler was next admitted a year later, initially as an in-patient for eight weeks, and then for 20 months as a day patient. His history from the start of his illness up to his discharge as it was then obtained is summarized below.

Revised history of presenting complaint

Mr Butler had first noticed that he was hard of hearing at the age of 20. This had not incommoded him until, as a result of promotion, he moved to a new open plan office in which there was a constant buzz of conversation. He had difficulty in hearing what was said to him, and social encounters became more and more of a strain. He took to drinking at lunch-time before going back to the office, and began to think that, not only was he being discussed by the young girls in the office, but that they were discussing his sexual inadequacy and indeed assumed that he was homosexual. He became preoccupied with his lack of previous sexual relationships and felt guilty about his previous sexual deviations, for which he thought he could be prosecuted. He gradually became convinced that he *was* going to be prosecuted for sexual offences and that the police were collecting evidence. His arrest for drunkenness reinforced this belief.

Mr Butler's mood gradually became depressed as his difficulties at work increased but he also came to feel more and more 'cornered' by the police and it is this which probably led to his suicide attempt. Both these feelings improved during his first two hospital admissions but Mr Butler could not face going back to work, and he resigned. He obtained another, less responsible, job but after 10 months became convinced that situations at work were being set up by the police to test him, his drinking increased and finally he left. He was unemployed for some time and gradually felt less 'cornered' by the police. However, he spent an increasing amount of time in bed. Eventually he took another job but this lasted less time than the first and was closely followed by several other short-term jobs until he was again charged with being drunk and disorderly. After this Mr Butler stayed at home and was frightened to go out because 'the police are everywhere putting pressure on me'.

Mr Butler discharged himself during his third admission because he believed that the hospital staff were in league with the police.

The admission during which the original history was obtained occurred some three months later. Mr Butler was treated with eight applications of electro-convulsive treatment (ECT), mianserin, and trifluoperazine during this period. His mental state improved considerably but it was not ascertained which of the three treatments was the most effective. He was not fully recovered on discharge: for example, Mr Butler thought that, although the police were no longer investigating him, they had done so in the past and may do so again.

Mr Butler was maintained in out-patients on imipramine and trifluoperazine. After four months he found a job in an accounts department and said that he was enjoying it despite having difficulty concentrating. However, three months later an elective left stapedectomy was performed following which his left ear was temporarily plugged and neuroleptics withdrawn in the general hospital. He became convinced that the nurses were treating him particularly coldly, and that this was because he had insulted some nurses in a public house some years before.

His suspicion of the police also returned after his discharge and a few days after returning to work he walked off the job. His medication was restarted and two months later Mr Butler was much less concerned about the police and work was again going well. His medication was gradually withdrawn by the psychiatrist who was following him up because he was thought to have recovered. However, his suspicions flared up again, he began drinking regularly at lunch-time and in the evenings, and subsequently he left his job. Trifluoperazine was restarted and Mr Butler felt well enough to get a temporary job. From the day that he started he was sure that his colleagues knew of the police's interest in him, and he only just managed to finish his two-week stint. A fortnight at another factory was even worse. Mr Butler's feelings of persecution fluctuated in intensity over the next two months. He was restarted on mianserin, and was slightly better after both his mianserin and his trifluoperazine were increased. One month later he felt himself to be as persecuted by the police and as guilty about his sexual misdemeanours as before, and 'on the brink of an overdose'. He was briefly admitted to hospital and was somewhat better on discharge, but still suspicious.

During the next few months Mr Butler spent more and more

time in bed. He refused day patient attendance but eventually wrote to the psychiatrist to describe the 'latest examples of police harassment' which included wiring his home to amplify the noise of traffic. He had taken, he wrote, to carrying a hammer to 'defend myself'. He was again admitted. The admitting psychiatrist noted that he was 'relaxed, not elated or depressed' even though he believed that the inverview was being recorded by agents of the police. No account of abnormal experiences was elicited.

Mr Butler's suspicions lessened on regular treatment with intramuscular depôt fluphenazine but he was noted to be withdrawn. He was referred to a day hospital where the admitting psychiatrist noted that, except for his ready smile, his face was unusually immobile and his tone of voice monotonous. His answers to questions were unusually non-discursive. Mr Butler rarely volunteered new information, and was noted never to initiate conversations with other patients.

Mr Butler was continued on intramuscular medication throughout his rehabilitation. He was very capable, particularly at clerical work, and was therefore given the patients' wages to prepare. However in his first week of this he became convinced that a fellow-patient was a plain-clothes policeman.

His suspicions subsided and four months later he was transferred to a vocational resettlement unit where he was noted to be a conscientious worker but unusually slow and lacking in initiative. His suspiciousness was also remarked upon, and indeed, during this time Mr Butler became increasingly convinced that there was a conspiracy against him to get information for the police or to test his masculinity—his account varied on different occasions. Eventually he refused to attend and he was referred to a day centre. At first he came in very late and often missed days without notice, but his attendance gradually became more regular. He had several minor relapses, usually after being given more responsibility. One paranoid episode began in a pub after an unusually heavy bout of drinking when he believed that a woman who asked him for a light was testing his virility. Fortunately, these relapses were successfully managed with a temporary increase in medication and a reassessment of his work programme.

Mr Butler became engaged to a fellow-patient about one year after starting at the day centre and, after an initial period of impotence began a regular sexual relationship with his fiancée.

Mental state examination (18 months after arrival at the day centre)

Appearance and general behaviour

Mr Butler was a markedly plump man who made no spontaneous movements. He had a mild Parkinsonian tremor when anxious. His voice was soft but normally modulated. His face was immobile except for occasional, self-deprecating smiles. His clothes were slightly unkempt and grubby.

Talk

His talk was unforthcoming about himself except that often at the end of an interview, he would ask whether he was getting better.

Mood

Mr Butler was slightly tense but not depressed. He described himself as feeling 'fine' in himself. He was attempting to diet to reduce weight.

Thought content

He was not at this time thinking much about the police although sometimes, when he remembered what had happened to him, he thought it 'funny' but did not like to think about it further. Mr Butler's mind quite often appeared to be empty of any thoughts.

Abnormal beliefs and interpretation of events

Very occasionally he experienced an everyday scene as being of special significance to him but he paid little attention to it and quickly forgot it.

Abnormal experiences

None were elicited.

Cognitive state

Mr Butler's orientation, memory, concentration and attention were all normal.

Appraisal of illness

He thought that he had an illness but that his present inability to reacclimatize to a work routine, was due to 'laziness'.

Summary

Mr Butler is a 39-year-old man with a 15-year history of a progressively more incapacitating tendency to ideas of reference and persecutory beliefs which have rendered him recently incapable of open employment.

The main challenge facing the psychiatrist treating Mr Butler at this stage is to minimize the frequency of relapse of his illness. A first step in meeting this challenge is to formulate the aetiology of relapse and to formulate possible prevention, or at least pre-emptive intervention.

Reformulation

Diagnosis

Mr Butler's gradual social deterioration, punctuated by episodes typical of the 'positive' symptoms of schizophrenia, makes the diagnosis of schizophrenia certain. Persecutory ideas continue to predominate so that paranoid schizophrenia remains the correct sub-type.

Aetiology

These also have become rather clearer. Mr Butler's deafness in combination with his lifelong shyness and social difficulties probably contributed to the development of his schizophrenia as it did to his relapse when one ear was occluded following a stapedectomy. However, effective treatment of his deafness has not arrested the progress of his illness.

Mr Butler is a regular heavy drinker. He uses alcohol to lower some of his social inhibitions, and, as indicated by his heavy drinking at least at the start of his illness, to try and reduce his fear of imaginary persecution. Although there has been at least one occasion when heavy drinking precipitated the development of a persecutory delusion which took some time to fade away, his normal steady intake appears not to exacerbate his illness.

The most important precipitants of relapse now seem to be first, the expectation of an authority (such as the manager of the day centre) that he take on more responsible work, and secondly, withdrawal of his medication. However, expectations placed on him by his family, and his fiancée may also be contributory factors.

Further investigations

The major outstanding investigation is to see Mr Butler with his parents.

Management

Mr Butler's long-term management has two goals: to minimize the dislocation and distress of relapse into positive symptoms, and help him to attain as normal work and social relationships as possible.

Regular out-patient follow-up is relevant to both these goals. The minimum dose of regular neuroleptic medication needs to be found which will keep his symptoms in abeyance. There also needs to be a pathway for him, his family and the manager at the day centre to the doctor so that a rapid increase in medication can be given if this is needed, for example, during a relapse of positive symptoms.

Out-patient sessions should also be used to encourage him to undertake the appropriate amount of work and domestic activity, and to monitor his progress in achieving his goals in these areas. Mr Butler is helped by encouragement and by being given a rationale for the treatment. The manager at the day centre (and, possibly in the future, the family) can also be encouraged to maintain a realistic expectation of Mr Butler's achievement and helped in their disappointment if he fails to achieve his goals.

A diet should be prescribed for him by the nutritionist as his increasing weight may predispose him to medical problems and can only exacerbate his social anxiety. As medication may have contributed to this, there is a further reason for keeping it to a minimum. Fluphenazine is no more likely than other neuroleptics to increase appetite, and a change of neuroleptics is therefore unlikely to be helpful.

Regular monitoring for the appearance of side-effects, particularly tardive dyskinesia, should be instituted. Anticholinergic agents often given, unnecessarily, to treat the side-effects of long-term neuroleptics should be avoided as they may increase the risk of dyskinesia.

Prognosis

Mr Butler is likely to remain socially disabled, although it can be expected that he will be free of his persecutory ideas most of the time. His mother has continued to supervise his appearance and self-care at home and provided him with meals and clean clothes. He will probably continue to need some degree of daily supervision of this kind. He is unlikely to obtain open employment and would become socially isolated if he were not pressed to attend a day centre.

The course of his illness cannot be predicted, but further deterioration can probably be prevented by the social treatments already mentioned. The risk of more severe deterioration is less than if Mr Butler had developed schizophrenia when he was younger, had not successfully established himself at work, and had a sub-type of schizophrenia other than 'paranoid'.

Postscript

Mr and Mrs Butler senior eventually agreed to be seen with their son. Both expressed their grief at their son's deterioration. No-one liked to talk about it at home. Mrs Butler's attitude to her son was critical but she was rarely firm with him for example about his helping out at home, or getting out of bed. Mr Butler kept out of his son's way. In an emotional moment he explained that if he behaved in a more concerned way he was afraid that his son would think that he was being treated as 'less than a man'.

Both were very frightened when the doctor spoke of their son as 'disabled', but they also seemed relieved.

Possibly the most useful result of this meeting, which was not repeated, was that Mr Butler subsequently discussed his father's relentless appetite for work. When he retired on medical grounds his father had taken another job straight away which entailed him getting up at 4.30 a.m. It was his son's inability to work that he and his son found so incomprehensible and disturbing about his illness. Mr Butler's wish to emulate his father seemed to explain Mr Butler's tendency to take on work which was beyond him, and then to react to the consequent stress by becoming more and more convinced that he was being persecuted.

11

A sudden attack of severe anxiety the case of Mrs Woolfe, aged 33

Presenting complaint

Five weeks before her referral to the psychiatry out-patient department, Mrs Woolfe, while driving to work, experienced a sudden attack of severe anxiety. She described an initial feeling of foreboding followed by the rapid development of extreme fear, which was accompanied by sweating, palpitations, choking sensations and difficulty in breathing. The episode lasted about an hour. Since that time she had suffered many similar attacks, averaging between two and three a day. Between episodes she was left feeling 'flat', tired, and drained. During the past three weeks she had, in addition, begun to feel low in spirits and lacking in energy. She found herself brooding on thoughts of death and had horrifying images of harming herself or those close to her. She felt that her life was now hopeless and that there was nothing to live for. Her sleep was very disturbed and she had lost one stone (6 kg) in weight. Her concentration had become so impaired that she had stopped working two weeks earlier. Diazepam 2 mg three times a day was prescribed by her general practitioner one week after the onset of her symptoms and this had provided some mild relief.

Mrs Woolfe attended with her cohabitee.

Family history

Mrs Woolfe's father, aged 72, was a retired schoolmaster. The patient described him as one of the healthiest people she had known until the previous year when he had suffered a myocardial infarct. Her father had a good physical recovery, but this episode left him preoccupied with his health.

The patient's mother, aged 60, had suffered 'from nerves' all

213

her life. Mrs Woolfe said that she could not recall her ever being completely 'well'. She always seemed to be tense, preoccupied with trivial worries, and frequently very low in spirits. She had also often complained of physical symptoms but her general practitioner was never able to make a clear-cut diagnosis of a physical illness. The usual treatment he prescribed for her was bed rest. Mother had always resisted referral to a psychiatrist despite frequent suggestions by her general practitioner. Six months before the patient's presentation her mother had suffered a cerebro-vascular accident and after some speech and motor impairment had now fully recovered.

The patient was the only child. The family was an extremely religious one; church was attended three times on Sundays and it was regarded as virtuous to forego all pleasures. The parents' marriage was always very secure and conflict was rare. Mother was the dominant partner. Despite a very strict upbringing the patient had always felt close to both parents and remembered always feeling that she must not hurt them. People had, from an early age, commented on her overdeveloped sense of guilt when acting not in accordance with her parents' wishes. Mother had an uncle who committed suicide. The patient knew no details about this as the matter was never discussed in the family. There was no other family history of mental illness.

Personal history

Mrs Woolfe's birth and early development were normal and her early childhood unremarkable. She commenced school, aged five, and there were some initial problems in settling down. She was reluctant to attend at first and on two or three occasions ran home. Her mother took her back immediately on each occasion and she soon became a happy primary school pupil. From the ages of eight to 16 years she attended a private school and passed eight O Levels. She made close friendships and was regarded by her teachers as a serious, hard-working girl. When she was 17 years old, she was sent to a new school to study for her A Levels. This school was very different from her previous one and she felt very unhappy there. She made no friends and was very upset by the fiercely competitive atmosphere. At this time she developed a number of symptoms (described under

Past psychiatric history). Despite these difficulties she gained three A Levels. Although she could have probably obtained university entrance Mrs Woolfe chose to go to a secretarial college. After qualifying she worked as a secretary in a building society's legal department where she impressed the staff with her abilities and after a year there she began to work for a firm of solicitors where again she showed herself to be an extremely capable person. However, after two years she left to raise her family, and she did not work again for five years.

She began working again seven years previously—this time at the head office of a publishing firm. Rapid promotion followed and at the time of her presentation she was in a senior managerial post bearing considerable responsibilities for organization and some of the legal aspects of the business. A month before the onset of her symptoms she had organized a large conference, which had been a strain.

In addition, she had commenced an external university degree course which she had done for two years.

The patient met her future husband when she was 16 years old. He was then 26, and a stockbroker, and they married three years later. They remained married for 13 years until Mrs Woolfe left her husband one year ago. There were two children, a boy, aged 11, and a girl, aged eight. Within a year or two of the marriage Mrs Woolfe began to feel that she had made a mistake. She described her husband as an overbearing man who would never discuss things with her on an equal standing. Although he had wanted to have children he spent little time with them. She tried unsuccessfully to tell him of her dissatisfaction and she suggested that they attend a marriage counsellor. This provoked arguments and he flatly refused to attend, even after she told him of an affair. On occasions he had been violent, although he never caused serious harm.

The couple finally separated, fairly amicably, one year previously. Mrs Woolfe went to live with her current cohabitant, Peter. He worked as an editor for the same firm as she and they had known each other for six years. They had decided simultaneously to leave their spouses, he proving more reluctant initially than she. Her children lived with them but Peter's daughter was with her mother. About two months prior to Mrs Woolfe's attendance at the hospital, Peter began to feel miserable, particularly about his limited access to his son. He told the patient that he had doubts about whether he could really love anyone again and decided that he would leave for two weeks to 'think it over'. It was after the first week that Mrs Woolfe developed her symptoms. Peter returned immediately and stated that his doubts were entirely resolved and that he wanted to carry on living with her.

Previous personality

Mrs Woolfe was normally an energetic woman. She was efficient, orderly, and reliable. She set high standards for herself which she rarely felt she achieved. Although she was sociable and friendly, she did not have any close friends apart from Peter. She coped well with strangers in the work environment. Many people commented on her life-long tendency to devalue herself and to blame herself if others were unhappy. Although not religious she had a high moral code of behaviour. At times she felt miserable, but apart from one occasion (see below) this had not interfered with her ability to cope. She was not an excessive worrier. She had many interests including music, especially ballet, and collected antique ceramics. She drank socially and was a non-smoker.

Past medical history

There was no significant previous physical illness.

Past psychiatric history

Although Mrs Woolfe had never seen a psychiatrist before, she described the development of clear-cut psychiatric symptoms when she was 17 years old. This occurred when she changed school to do her A Levels. During a play-reading at school she developed her first attack of severe anxiety, the features of which were identical to those described this time. She went on to develop a number of phobic symptoms as well, particularly of crowded places, buses, and shops. These had become so intense that she was unable to attend school for about six weeks. Gradually, with the help of her general practitioner and her parents, who encouraged her to go out, she improved, although the symp-

toms were present altogether for about one year. During that
time she recalled feeling quite depressed.

Since that time she had, however, remained almost completely
symptom-free apart from occasional apprehension of travelling
on the underground.

Mental state examination

Appearance and general behaviour

Mrs Woolfe was a petite, slim lady who, when the interview commenced, said that she was too anxious to speak and suggested
that Peter be called in to give an account of her problems. She
appeared very anxious and complained of sweating palms and of
a feeling of breathlessness. At times she was tearful, particularly
when describing her more distressing symptoms.

Talk

After some initial reassurance she was able to give a well organized and fluent account of herself and required little prompting.

Mood

She described a depressed mood. She felt 'worn out', 'incompetent' and 'hopeless'—'however hard I try I'm just not going to
get better . . . there's just a terrible, terrible sadness—a sort of
continual hurt inside'. On direct questioning she admitted to
some fleeting suicidal thoughts but she did not feel that things
had reached that point 'yet'. She had no appetite and had lost
over a stone (6 kg) in weight in five weeks. Her sleep was also
poor with initial insomnia and early morning waking (3 or 4
a.m.). She described a marked diurnal variation in her mood,
feeling at her worst first thing in the morning and better by the
early afternoon. Her depressed mood was sustained without
even a moment's relief and she found no pleasure in anything.

Thought content

A number of preoccupations emerged. She was terrified of her
panic attacks. These consisted of an intense experience of fear
and were accompanied by the somatic symptoms previously
described. She feared that she might die during one of these
attacks. She also described extremely distressing, vivid, stereo-

typed, recurrent images, usually of harming herself or those close to her, such as stabbing herself with a kitchen knife. She attempted to push these intrusive images out of her mind and she feared that she might act them out although she did not wish to. Mrs Woolfe also described a number of guilt-laden ruminations, particularly about having abandoned her husband and about being a burden on her parents and Peter. She said that she had let her parents down badly although conceding that they had supported her separation from her husband and that they liked Peter. She denied any fears now that Peter would leave her and she described him in the kindest terms.

No current phobic symptoms were elicited.

Abnormal beliefs and interpretation of events

No delusions or hallucinations were elicited. Her ideas of guilt and hopelessness were not of delusional intensity and she had no hypochondriacal preoccupations.

Abnormal experiences

Mrs Woolfe described no abnormal experiences, in particular no symptoms of depersonalization.

Cognitive state

Cognitive testing revealed her to be well orientated and without any signs of memory impairment. She was able to concentrate well enough to perform 'serial sevens' without difficulty, although she had complained that her concentration was impaired to the extent that she could not look at a newspaper nor watch even a short television programme.

Appraisal of illness

She could not readily accept that she was ill and at one point said that there was nothing that could change her, and, therefore, she was wasting the doctor's valuable time. 'There are surely many more needy people than me—the responsibility for my state lies with me'.

Physical examination

The general practitioner had performed a physical examination before referring Mrs Woolfe to the psychiatrist and this had revealed no abnormality.

Peter was seen after Mrs Woolfe had been interviewed. He confirmed the history in every detail and described her personality before her illness in similar terms to her own description.

Summary

Mrs Woolfe is a 33-year-old woman who has separated from her husband and recently had a brief separation from her cohabitant. Following this she has felt panicky, anxious, and more recently, depressed. This type of problem is frequently met in out-patients, where the psychiatrist needs to reach a clear diagnosis in order to start treatment. In Mrs Woolfe's case the important diagnostic issues are whether her symptoms reflect primarily a depressive or anxiety-based disturbance, and whether such a disturbance should be accepted as a 'normal' response situation.

Formulation

Diagnosis

In descriptive terms Mrs Woolfe's presentation was dominated by symptoms of anxiety and depression. The major possibilities to be considered are: a depressive illness, an anxiety state or an adjustment reaction.

Most of the symptoms typical of an anxiety state were present. These included subjective anxiety with somatic accompaniments (sweating, palpitations, choking sensations, difficulty in breathing) which often occur in typical panic attacks. The anxiety was diffuse and not focused on any particular situation or object. The short duration of the symptoms is also consistent with this diagnosis. However, there were also a number of depressive symptoms which were severe in intensity and which tended to dominate the mental state examination. An admixture of depressive symptoms in patients with an anxiety state is common but these are not generally as marked as in this case. The onset of an anxiety state is usually, but not always, in association with a precipitating factor. In this case, the departure of Mrs Woolfe's cohabitant to think about their relationship coincided with the onset of her symptoms.

The presence of clear-cut depressive symptoms leads to a consideration of a depressive illness as the primary diagnosis. The symptoms in Mrs Woolfe's case are: a sustained depressed mood, lack of energy, poor concentration, a feeling of hopelessness that she will ever change, ideas of guilt about abandoning her husband, of letting down her parents, of being a burden on those she loves and of being responsible for her current state and therefore of wasting the psychiatrist's time. She also had the so-called 'biological' features of depression—appetite disturbance and weight loss, early morning waking and diurnal mood variation. In addition she admitted to fleeting suicidal ideas. The terrifying visual images of harming herself or others are obsessional in nature, in that they were unwanted, intrusive, stereotyped mental contents which she attempted to resist and which she perceived as alien to her personality and inappropriate. Their content was morbid and depressive. Obsessional symptoms of this type are common in depressive illnesses. Anxiety symptoms are also common in depressive illness although they do not usually stand out as starkly as in this case. The combination of depression and tension in Mrs Woolfe might warrant a description of agitated depression.

The third possibility to be considered is an 'adjustment reaction'. This is a mild or transient disturbance which is usually closely related in time and content to an obvious stressful event. Mrs Woolfe's symptoms developed in close relationship to Peter leaving. However, the extent of her disturbance and its failure to improve when Peter returned, suggests that this was more than an adjustment reaction. With time her symptoms of depression had in fact intensified. Furthermore, the content of her depressive and anxious preoccupations were not directly related to the separation. An element which should be considered in addition to the 'stress' is a person's vulnerability to this type of stress. Here it should be noted that Mrs Woolfe had suffered psychological distress twice before, at times of major changes in her life. The first, when she started school was apparently mild and transient, whilst the second when she went to her A level school was prolonged, severe and comprised a mixture again of depression and anxiety symptoms, in the latter case taking the form of panic attacks and agoraphobia. The second episode, as in the present illness, appears to have been too long-lived and severe to be termed an adjustment reaction. Between the ages of 18 and 33 Mrs Woolfe coped well with many stresses with no evidence of major disruptions of her life.

Overall, the most likely diagnosis is of a depressive illness. A common difficulty in classifying depression into 'reactive' or 'neurotic' on the one hand or 'endogenous' or 'psychotic' on the other is exemplified here as the illness has the features of both. Although there appears to be a precipitant and anxiety symptoms are prominent, there are also many features of an 'endogenous' depression, such as early morning waking, more severe depression in the morning and strong feelings of guilt.

There is the possibility that this is Mrs Woolfe's second depressive illness, the first having occurred when she was 17 years old.

Aetiology

There is a family history of mental disorder. Mrs Woolfe's mother has had life-long problems of a psychological kind, possibly with depressive and anxiety symptoms. Also, her mother's uncle committed suicide, raising the possibility that he might have suffered from a severe depressive illness. The transmission of a psychiatric disorder from mother to daughter could be by genetic or learning influences or a combination of both.

In the year prior to the development of her illness, Mrs Woolfe experienced an astonishing number of stressful life events. She left her husband to live with another man, her father had a heart attack, her mother had a stroke, she was promoted at work, and finally Peter left home. There is a relationship between life events and the onset of illnesses of many kinds. In general the type of life event does not have a specific relationship with the type of illness which ensues although 'losses' defined broadly are often associated with depressive symptoms. Usually the type of illness which develops bears a closer relationship to the patient's particular vulnerabilities which in turn are linked to 'constitutional' factors (in which genetics, for example, may play a role), and past experiences.

Mrs Woolfe is an intelligent and capable woman who from the information available appears to be of a reasonably stable disposition, at least since her late teens. There are, however, some aspects of her personality which might have made some of the life changes she experienced specially difficult for her to manage. A theme running through her life has been a special sensitivity to her very religious parents and a propensity for feeling guilty if others should feel disappointed or unhappy. Her parents had a strict code of conduct and Mrs Woolfe expressed a loyalty to it. Leaving her husband to live with another man followed by the development of serious illnesses in both parents might be expected to affect Mrs Woolfe with special force. Peter's leaving may then have spelled the final disappointment and sign of failure in re-establishing her life which might have made amends for leaving her husband. Less important, although possibly of significance, might have been her rapid promotion at work, which entailed new responsibilities. This might have proved very stressful for a person like Mrs Woolfe whose high standards, conscientiousness and need to be in control, although not extreme, are judged to be greater than normal. These life-long perfectionist traits are not sufficiently prominent in the patient to merit a description of an 'obsessional' personality.

The content of many of Mrs Woolfe's preoccupations in her illness can be seen to derive from some of the central themes in her life: guilt at letting others down, being a burden on her close ones, harming her close ones, incompetence.

Further investigations

At this stage there is sufficient information to make a diagnosis and to plan the initial treatment, especially since Peter has been interviewed and has confirmed the history as given by Mrs Woolfe.

It would be useful to know more about the family history of mental disorder and whether her mother and her mother's uncle had suffered from depressive illness. The family doctor might be able to provide useful information here.

The stability of Mrs Woolfe's relationship with Peter and their hopes for the future need some exploration and this could be done in a joint session with the couple. It is not clear that seeing Mrs Woolfe's parents at this stage would add any important information.

Management

Mrs Woolfe presents with a moderately severe depressive illness which may still be getting worse. The question of admission to hospital needs to be considered, particularly as she has entertained some suicidal thoughts and will need considerable supervision and support.

During the interview Mrs Woolfe eventually made a good rapport and she appeared to speak openly about her feelings with no attempt at concealment. Peter expressed a wish to look after her and they both agreed that Mrs Woolfe's parents could also be enlisted to help. Admission may thus not be necessary. It is important at this stage to explain to Mrs Woolfe and Peter that she is suffering from a depressive illness and that she will almost certainly recover from this. It might also prove helpful to reassure her about the nature of some of her symptoms: that she will not die from her panic attacks and that she will not act on her obsessional impulses. To be effective, explanation and reassurance require the establishment of a good doctor–patient relationship and his must be an immediate and major goal.

Antidepressant medication is indicated in this case. Amitriptyline would be suitable because it also has sedative effects. The anticipated delay in the response to medication should be mentioned, as should possible side-effects. In view of the seriousness of the illness she should be seen weekly initially, in order to monitor the effectiveness of the medication, to intervene if her condition should deteriorate and to provide continuing support for her and Peter until she improves.

The longer-term management will depend on Mrs Woolfe's response to medication. It is to be expected that she will improve over the next month or so. As long as her improvement is maintained simple psychological support should suffice. If significant problems in her relationship with Peter emerge these might be tackled in joint interviews when the depression has improved.

Prognosis

The prognosis for recovery from this episode is excellent. The acute onset with clear-cut depressive symptoms marking a radical change from the patient's normal self augur a good response to medication. Mrs Woolfe is a woman with many personality assets and she should be able to resume her normal life. There remains the possibility that she may have further episodes of depression, particularly as this may now be her second illness. Such an episode is most likely to occur if she is exposed to mounting pressures.

Brief formulation

Mrs Woolfe is a 33-year-old, separated mother of two, who has cohabited with another man for the past year. She has a high-level managerial post in a large firm. Five weeks previously she developed panic attacks with subjective feelings of intense fear and with somatic accompaniments. Over the same period of time she has felt depressed, lacking in energy, hopeless, with some guilty ruminations and disturbing, violent, visual images. When she was 17, she suffered for about a year from panic attacks, agoraphobic symptoms and depressive symptoms. She made an almost complete recovery from these and was well until the onset of her current symptoms.

Diagnosis

The most likely diagnosis is a depressive illness in view of her prominent and clear-cut depressive symptoms which include 'biological' ones—weight loss, early morning waking and diurnal mood variation. The visual images are obsessional in nature.

The presence of marked anxiety symptoms, particularly at the onset, raises the question of whether this is primarily an anxiety state. However, such symptoms are frequently found in a depressive illness and in this case they are less prominent than the depressive ones.

An 'adjustment reaction' is unlikely in view of the severity of her disturbance, her failure to improve when her separation from

Peter ended and the fact that the content of her preoccupations was not directly related to this precipitating factor.

Aetiology

There is a family history of mental disorder, which may indicate a genetic factor. In the year prior to her illness Mrs Woolfe had experienced a number of major life events—separation from her husband, illness in both parents and promotion at work. Peter's leaving home was an obvious precipitating event. Mrs Woolfe's personality also played a role, particularly her sensitivity to her parents' expectations, her high moral standards, her tendency towards guilt, her conscientiousness and her need to be in control of situations.

Further investigations

There is sufficient information to make a diagnosis and plan the initial treatment. More details of the family history of mental disorder would be useful. The stability of Mrs Woolfe's relationship with Peter needs further exploration.

Management

Although Mrs Woolfe is moderately depressed the absence of active suicidal ideation and the presence of good social supports makes admission unnecessary. A good doctor–patient relationship and some reassurance on a number of points of her condition are important. Antidepressant medication is indicated as is weekly follow-up to monitor her progress and to provide further support. Longer-term plans will depend upon her response to treatment.

Prognosis

Mrs Woolfe's symptoms should improve with medication and support, but the risk of recurrence in the future is considerable.

Further information

Following discussion along the lines mentioned under the management above, Mrs Woolfe indicated that she would be prepared to take medication although she did not see that it could possibly help.

Over the next three months she did well. She was seen weekly initially and then fortnightly. The dose of amitriptyline was increased to 50 mg three times a day and her depressive and anxiety symptoms markedly diminished. Peter appeared concerned and supportive. Problems between the couple were consistently denied, and evidence of their existence did not emerge in two joint sessions. After six weeks absence, Mrs Woolfe returned to work. She was somewhat lacking in confidence but managed to cope well. After three months she was discharged from the clinic. She remained somewhat troubled by very occasional panic attacks and the fear that her depression might recur. Her general practitioner was advised to continue her medication for another three months and then to tail it off.

However, nine months after her original presentation Mrs Woolfe was referred back to the clinic. Many of her symptoms had recurred but had not reached their previous intensity. Amitriptylene had been stopped two months previously. Two new events had occurred—the offer of a divorce from her husband and the need to organize a large conference for her firm.

The psychiatrist decided that Mrs Woolfe was having a relapse of her depressive illness, probably because her medication had been stopped prematurely. However, on this occasion another observation was made. Although Mrs Woolfe responded strikingly to reassurance from the doctor, Peter seemed unable to comfort her at all. In addition whenever the subject of the couple's relationship was raised by the psychiatrist, particularly any reference to Peter's leaving, it was always avoided by a shift to another topic. At these times Mrs Woolfe and Peter looked away from each other. There was a sense that all was not well with the couple. It was decided, therefore, to see them together for a few sessions to understand this more.

Amitriptyline was recommenced and again Mrs Woolfe improved gradually. During the joint sessions it was striking how protective of each other the couple were. They seemed at pains not to distress each other and hints of disagreement, when taken up by the doctor, were quickly detoured to a discussion of Mrs Woolfe's symptoms. At times Peter uttered some quite depressive thoughts, mainly concerning his son whom he felt he had let down by leaving his wife. These were quickly covered up, usually by Mrs Woolfe saying this was understandable and only temporary.

Three months after Mrs Woolfe's return to the clinic she came alone. She had been unable to persuade Peter to come and reported that he had become listless, uncommunicative, and ruminated excessively about his son. He was unwilling to discuss his feelings with her. She admitted for the first time that these spells had occurred frequently, particularly in the first six months of their cohabitation. At these times she felt helpless in her attempts to influence his mood. She was encouraged by the doctor to try again to bring Peter back next time.

The next time Mrs Woolfe came with a friend. Peter had left her and gone to live with his parents. Peter's wife had remarried and he had become extremely depressed. He had also expressed some vague persecutory idea concerning people at work. Mrs Woolfe's friend said that Peter had been inclined to depressive moods all along and that Mrs Woolfe had struggled continuously to prop him up. Mrs Woolfe admitted for the first time that she had been very concerned about Peter, even from the commencement of their cohabitation. There had been weekends when Peter stayed in bed for practically the entire time, not bothering to wash or eat and was 'engrossed in his own thoughts to which he denied me access'. On one occasion he expressed some bizarre ideas about the bedroom light which he felt in some way was 'spying' on his thoughts and behaviour. Mrs Woolfe had 'hugged him like a child to comfort him'. In the view of her friend, the couple had never succeeded in establishing a sense of 'family' in the household.

Although Mrs Woolfe was distressed by Peter leaving, there was a quality, different in kind, from her previous state of depression. Her reaction appeared normal. In fact, it seemed as if a burden had been eased. It became clear how troubling the relationship had been to her, particularly Peter's imperviousness to her attempts to make him feel better. She was someone who needed to see her efforts rewarded in order to feel worthwhile. Her sense of loyalty to him had prevented her from disclosing this earlier.

Although Peter has left Mrs Woolfe following her relapse, she seems to have improved. The context of her depression has now changed and the psychiatrist needs to modify his original formulation in order to take account of this. In particular, he will need to understand more fully why she first became depressed in order to develop further lines of treatment.

Reformulation

Diagnosis

The original diagnosis remains depression. Mrs Woolfe has suffered a subsequent relapse, but has now improved.

Aetiology

It seems possible that the withdrawal of medication contributed to Mrs Woolfe's relapse. Her first episode of depression, when she was 17, had lasted for one year. The psychiatrist's advice about when to discontinue medication had not taken into account the possibility that this might have been the natural time course of her illness.

Mrs Woolfe had also been given responsibility for organizing another conference. A similar event occurred a month before she first became depressed and it seems likely that this stress also contributed as a trigger to her relapse.

Although the offer of a divorce from her husband might have been expected and also what she wanted, it would also have been stressful—not only because it finalized their separation, but also because of its impact upon her relationship with Peter. For one thing she would be in a position to remarry and might feel emotional pressure to do so. In the light of what has been discovered about Peter this would have been a considerable source of worry.

Peter's seriously disturbed behaviour was obviously an important factor contributing to Mrs Woolfe's depression. The fact that she was living with him was presumably a continuous source of stress and since this was never revealed to the psychiatrist, he was unable to provide any counselling about it. Both Peter and Mrs Woolfe had actively avoided bringing his problem to the psychiatrist in spite of ample encouragement, which seems surprising considering the strain it must have imposed upon their relationship. Although Peter might have been reluctant to discuss this because he was feeling persecuted, there may have been reasons for Mrs Woolfe to avoid this issue also.

Her sense of guilt when others are unhappy might have made her feel that she must try and sort out Peter's problems on her own. Furthermore, there are similarities between Peter and the way she described her first husband. In particular they were both unable to share and work out problems with her as she would have liked. It is not uncommon for people to develop relationships with a recurring pattern of this nature which often seem to reflect some difficulty of their own. In Mrs Woolfe's case the fact that she felt that she had made the same mistake twice might have been sufficient reason for not drawing the psychiatrist's attention to it. There were also similarities between Mrs Woolfe's problem and Peter's, in particular their feeling of guilt about a broken marriage. It is again not uncommon for someone to find a partner with similar problems to their own.

These factors suggest how Mrs Woolfe might have been drawn into a distressing relationship with Peter and reasons why she might have found it difficult to discuss this with the psychiatrist. It now seems clearer how her depression developed and was maintained in the context of her relationship with Peter. It also seems likely that aspects of her personality made her particularly susceptible to develop such a relationship in the first place.

Further investigations

The likelihood that aspects of her personality have made Mrs Woolfe vulnerable to depression means that these need to be clarified. For example, it has been suggested that for some reason she develops relationships with men who are unable to discuss problems with her. She then seems to make a considerable effort to support them, whilst at the same time resenting their inability to share experiences with her. Once the psychiatrist has established that there are such recurring patterns in her relationships he would be able to find out whether she can reflect upon these. He might do this by clarifying ways in which she felt she might have contributed to any difficulties that existed between herself and Peter or her husband.

In this way the psychiatrist would be able to develop a clearer picture of Mrs Woolfe's vulnerability to depression. He would also be testing out her ability to make use of this information within the framework of a psychotherapeutic relationship.

Management

She will continue to require antidepressant medication because of the severity of her symptoms and their tendency to recur. These should be withdrawn under supervision only after she has made a sustained recovery. Increasing attention will be directed towards psychotherapeutic interventions, which will involve clarification of those issues which have been mentioned.

Prognosis

She again appears to have made a good recovery from the immediate episode. We would predict that she is vulnerable to relapse if she should make subsequent relationships of a similar nature, which will depend in part on her response to psychotherapy.

Postscript

The psychiatrist continued Mrs Woolfe's antidepressant medication and saw her every month in the out-patient department. Although Peter did not return she frequently talked about him. She also expressed considerable doubt about her ability to live without a man. The psychiatrist focused on her lack of self-confidence and responded by being supportive and reassuring. He reminded her of her strengths, whilst also providing her with the opportunity to discuss her self-doubt. She managed this transition competently and was surprised by her own resources as well as the support which was forthcoming from her parents and close friends. She carried on with her work and over the following year suffered no recurrence of her depressive symptoms.

12

A psychosomatic problem—the case of Mrs Joan Baker, aged 36

Presenting complaint

Mrs Baker was referred to the psychiatric out-patient department by her general practitioner for advice about her 'constant need to pass urine'. In his letter the general practitioner asked if this symptom could have been 'psychological'. He also mentioned that she recently had been examined by a urological surgeon who found no physical abnormality in her bladder. Mrs Baker attended her appointment with her husband. She was asked whether she wanted to be interviewed alone, but she replied she would prefer her husband to be with her. She then gave the following account of her symptoms.

She said that her bladder felt 'full' immediately after she urinated and that she was therefore continually preoccupied with going to the toilet. When she did pass urine, it was generally a small quantity. As far as she was concerned 'I do not know what it is like to go to the toilet and then not think about going anymore'. She attempted to control this feeling by 'trying to put it out of my mind', 'keeping busy', or 'willing it out', but none of these strategies had worked for any length of time. This preoccupation with emptying her bladder fluctuated in intensity, but on occasions led to her going to the toilet up to four times in half an hour, or over a dozen times during the daytime. She had not noticed any specific provocative situations, but had the impression that this feeling was worse in the mornings and improved when she was busily involved in doing something. However, Mrs Baker said that she was also anxious about leaving her home, because she felt she always had to be near a toilet and this made her cut down on doing things like shopping.

This 'problem' started suddenly, two and a half years previously. She could remember the exact occasion, a Sunday, immediately after dinner, but could remember nothing else being special about that day. Since that time, it had been a 'constant worry' which she was unable to eradicate from her mind. Her general practitioner had treated her with tricyclic antidepressants and she was currently taking amitriptyline 50 mg at night and flurazepam 30 mg at night. However, nothing produced any improvement in her symptoms.

She said that her general practitioner also referred her to another psychiatrist two years previously, as well as to the urological surgeon. The first psychiatrist who saw her admitted her to hospital for a fortnight.

Family history

Her father died 16 years previously of a myocardial infarct, when he was aged 45. He suffered his first heart attack 12 years before that, but refused to let this interfere with this life. He ignored his doctor's advice and continued to lead an active life, working regularly as a car salesman and enjoying fishing which was his main hobby. He had no further problems with his heart until the fatal episode, which occurred three months after his own father had died from a heart attack. Mrs Baker discovered her father's body within a few seconds of his death and remembered feeling 'frightened and helpless, not really knowing what was going on'. She found him collapsed on the stairs and ran to a neighbour's house to call an ambulance. By the time this arrived, her father was dead.

She said that she always felt very close to her father and considered him a warm, supportive, and caring man. She was very upset by his death and remembered feeling miserable for several months afterwards, during which time she dreamed about him frequently. These dreams had continued intermittently until the present time.

Her mother was aged 66 and was described as being generally 'miserable' since her husband died. Six years previously she also suffered a small heart attack which was treated at home. Since then she had experienced mild angina, which responded to medication. She lived a few miles from Mrs Baker and they maintained daily contact, either by meeting or speaking on the telephone. Her mother was also bothered by mild arthritis, which rarely required medication.

Mrs Baker was the youngest of three siblings. Her sister, who was four years older than herself, was married with two children. Her brother was two years older than herself and also married. She described her family as close and supportive and said that they still met regularly.

There was no family history of psychiatric illness.

Personal history

Mrs Baker was born in a small town in the north of England, where she spent all her life. She remembered her childhood as being a very happy one and had 'only very vague' memories about her father's first heart attack, which occurred when she was about eight. When she was asked whether she ever wet her bed as a child she said that as far as she knew she 'became dry' at the age of three and that this had never been a problem for her.

She never enjoyed school and made no close friends there. She attributed this to her general lack of interest in studying. She never achieved any formal qualifications and left school at the age of 15. When she was talking about school she spontaneously said that on the day that she left she cried and at the time she remembered thinking this was 'rather odd' since she had been looking forward to leaving.

After leaving school she became a catering assistant and remained working for the same firm until she was 19 years old. She then managed to get a promotion by moving to another firm, where she stayed until she was 26. She enjoyed this job considerably, but left because she married and became pregnant. Since that time she had no further employment outside the home and she said that she thoroughly enjoyed being a housewife.

Her menarche occurred when she was aged 16, at the same time she began going out with boys. She had three boyfriends before meeting her husband, Frank. Each of these relationships lasted for over a year, but none of them involved having sexual intercourse. She met Frank, who was three years older than herself, at her second job where he was employed as an electrician. They knew each other for three years before they married when she was 23. They had two children, Elizabeth aged nine and Leonard aged six, both of whom were described as 'healthy and normal'.

Leonard suffered from sleep problems for the first three years of his life and this was sufficiently worrying for him to have been referred to their general practitioner who prescribed regular night sedation.

Mr and Mrs Baker described their sexual relationship as 'satisfactory', but said that the frequency had fallen from four times to twice a week over the last year or so. They said that their marriage was a 'very happy one' and there were no financial problems. In fact they were very comfortably off and since their marriage Frank had built up a building firm of which he was the managing director.

Apart from looking after her family and maintaining regular contact with her mother, Mrs Baker had no active interests or social life. She said 'I found myself going out less in the evenings with Frank, because of my problem'.

Past medical history

Mrs Baker had a hysterectomy for menorrhagia six years previously. Following Leonard's birth she suffered increasingly heavy and prolonged menstrual bleeding, which she found very distressing. She attended her local hospital and was put on the waiting list for admission and investigation. However, this would have meant a delay of several months and because she felt unable to cope with this, she speeded up the process by seeing a private gynaecologist who performed a hysterectomy. As far as she knew the gynaecologist had left her ovaries intact and she said that she still experienced monthly 'changes' in herself (such as breast swelling and slight tension) which she had previously associated with her 'periods'.

Three months previously she was referred to the local urologist because of her urinary symptoms. He admitted her for two days for investigation and treatment. He told her that he found nothing wrong with her bladder but had performed a dilatation 'to see if it would help'.

Past psychiatric history

On direct questioning Mrs Baker said that five years previously she became very worried about her physical health, particularly the state of her heart, when she suffered from frequent 'palpitations'. At that time she felt considerable anxiety, cried practically all the time, lost 3 kg in weight and experienced sleep disturbance. Her general practitioner treated her with night sedation, which alleviated her symptoms, but did not eradicate them. It was the deterioration of these symptoms over a period of several weeks that led to her admission to the local psychiatric hospital two years previously. She said that at that time she had thoughts of harming herself.

She was admitted for two weeks and said that she was treated 'terribly'. She remembered being given exercises to help her relax and a tape to accompany these. She also said that she had to keep a record of when she felt the urge to pass urine. Although she said that her symptoms improved a little as a result of her treatment, she had been most affected by an episode when another patient made sexual advances to her. She felt 'the other patients made me worse'.

Previous personality

Both she and her husband agreed that she had always been a quiet, rather shy person who would 'keep things to myself'. She generally became upset easily, but never seemed to lose her temper, even when her children were being quite naughty. She tended to worry a great deal about them when they were out of her sight, particularly Leonard. She was also quite a meticulous person, particularly when it came to keeping the house tidy.

Mental state examination

Appearance and general behaviour

Mrs Baker was a tall, attractive brunette who was smartly and tidily dressed. She sat still with her hands clasped on the side of the chair throughout most of the interview but occasionally she glanced at her husband as if to ask for confirmation or clarification of some of her answers.

Talk

Her voice was hesitant and she only spoke in response to the questions the psychiatrist put to her or to his prompting. However, when she did reply her answers were coherent and detailed. Her husband often continued her answers when she paused. She would then agree with him and continue.

Mood

Mrs Baker looked sad, anxious, and frightened for most of the interview and on occasion, particularly when talking about her father, she seemed very close to tears. She also said that she felt 'guilty' about her problem because she believed that it might spoil her marriage. Her preoccupation with passing urine meant that she and Frank were unable to go out to the cinema or parties. In spite of this 'getting me down' she said that she had not become so upset that she felt life was not worth living and seemed quite shocked at the possibility that she might want to harm herself.

She said that her sleep had been intermittently disturbed over the last few years. Much of the time she found it difficult to fall asleep because she was worrying about her 'problem', but she also woke up early in the mornings and this had become more frequent recently. She was not enjoying her food and may have lost about 7 lb (3 kg) five years previously, but her weight was now steady.

Thought content

She was mainly preoccupied with her presenting symptoms of frequency and urgency, as described. She said that the was frightened that it might have a physical cause and although she felt partly reassured by the urologist's assessment, she remained a little uncertain about this.

There was no evidence of phobias.

Abnormal beliefs and interpretation of events

None were elicited.

Abnormal experiences

None were elicited.

Cognitive state

This was not formally tested since from the account that she gave of her illness there appeared to be no disturbance of her memory, intelligence or concentration.

Appraisal of illness

Mrs Baker agreed that she could be depressed but attributed this to her constant preoccupation with passing urine. However, she added that whatever the cause she was 'determined to get this problem treated'.

Physical examination

This was not performed because the general practitioner's letter said that Mrs Baker was physically fit and that all investigations were normal. Furthermore, the psychiatrist who examined her did not think there were any specific indications for a further examination.

Summary

Mrs Baker is a 36-year-old married woman who presents with a two and a half year history of urgency of micturition, which has failed to respond to both psychiatric and physical intervention. In this case the formulation will need to be directed towards elucidating the extent to which her symptoms could be attributed to a physical or a psychiatric disorder. This is the problem presented by the general practitioner, and its solution will clearly determine the management of this case.

Formulation

Diagnosis

The manner in which Mrs Baker presented her problem is characteristic of an obsession. She experienced her need to urinate as intrusive and she attempted to control it by using various psychological strategies. She tried to extinguish it by eradicating the thought or by involving herself in other activities. The fact that these strategies failed means that she felt compelled to empty her bladder, but only passed a small quantity of urine. However, this failed to deal effectively with the obsession which immediately returned, setting off once again the cycle of events.

There are several other features about her complaint which suggest strongly that it has important psychological components. Although Mrs Baker described discomfort in her bladder, she also located the problem in her mind. For example, she said she did 'not know what it is like to go to the toilet and then not *think* about going anymore'. She also tried to control this symptom by 'putting it out of my *mind*'.

Mrs Baker therefore presented her symptom as affecting the way she feels and thinks. These features might well have been influenced by her previous contact with a psychiatrist and the atmosphere that accompanies a psychiatric interview. Nevertheless, they are consistent with her problem having an important psychological aspect, even though it could still be associated with a primary, physical disturbance.

In addition to her symptoms having psychological characteristics Mrs Baker demonstrated many features of an affective disturbance. She looked miserable and tense, felt desperate about her situation and described other symptoms such as sleep disturbance, which had been present for several years. In fact, her history suggests that she has had symptoms of anxiety and depression for the previous six years and that she has also had previous hypochondriacal symptoms. Six years previously, following her son's birth, she had a hysterectomy for menorrhagia. Menorrhagia is not only an uncommon post-puerperal complication, but it may also be misdiagnosed on the basis of unsubstantiated complaints, particularly when a woman is depressed.

Five years previously she suffered a period of extreme anxiety and preoccupation with her health, for which her general practitioner prescribed a tricyclic antidepressant and offered reassurance. Following this her symptoms appeared to improve, although she said that Leonard then slept poorly for the first three years of his life and had to be treated with sedatives. In fact, her urinary symptoms appear to have started when Leonard's insomnia improved. Although it is impossible to ascribe a clear cause to this it would be reasonable to assume that being depressed made it difficult for her to look after Leonard and that this might have reflected itself in his sleep disturbance.

It therefore seems that Mrs Baker has a moderately severe affective disorder with features of both depression and anxiety, which has lasted for the last four to five years. Since a sense of urgency is a frequent accompaniment to anxiety, her presenting symptom can be explained by the presence of a psychiatric illness.

The fact that her urgency seems likely to be a psychiatric symptom does not exclude an underlying physical disorder, although in Mrs Baker's case there are several reasons why this seems to be unlikely. First, she had no other urological symptoms such as straining, pain or discomfort, which might be expected in a disorder causing such severe urgency. Secondly, Mrs Baker was physically well and had no evidence of any general illness such as diabetes mellitus, which might also cause these symptoms. Thirdly, all the investigations undertaken so far have proved normal.

Mrs Baker's symptoms can therefore be attributed to a psychiatric disorder for three reasons. First, she has clear manifestations of depression and anxiety; secondly, her symptoms have fundamental psychological characteristics; and thirdly, her history, examination, and investigation do not suggest that there is a significant physical disorder which can explain them.

Although Mrs Baker has marked features of anxiety, she presented these in the context of a clear depression. Over the last five years she seems to have had fairly persistent, although fluctuating affective symptoms. Many of these appear to have been anxiety related, but on at least one occasion she described a disturbance of sleep and appetite and at the very beginning she presented with marked physical symptoms. It is therefore unclear at the present time whether she has had a chronic depressive illness, or a chronic anxiety state with intermittent depression.

Aetiology

There are several factors that appear to have contributed to the development of Mrs Baker's depression. She first became unwell after Leonard was born and when her mother suffered a small myocardial infarct. This episode may have re-awoken memories of her father's death which were particularly painful and frightening for her not only because of their affection but because she was the first one to discover his body. Anxiety would be an expected reaction to such a severely threatening situation, and she was likely to have been particularly vulnerable to this during her puerperium.

Her difficulties would have been aggravated further by Leonard's insomnia, which required treatment by her general practitioner. She then began to complain of menorrhagia which was considered severe enough to justify a hysterectomy being performed. Although it is unclear whether she was having extremely heavy periods or whether her depressed mood lowered her threshold for complaint, the hysterectomy is itself likely to have been an additional stressful experience particularly in a woman who was only 31 years old.

Although these factors may explain why Mrs Baker first became depressed at this time, there seem to be other aspects of her personality which made her particularly vulnerable to developing a depression. Although her close relationship with her parents could be seen as a protective factor, the threat of losing her mother would have been particularly worrying. She also seems to have been a shy girl who made emotionally intense relationships which surprised even her. An example of this was her reaction to crying before she left school when she thought she was looking forward to it. This suggests that she was not 'psychologically-minded' which would have therefore made her less able to recognize and handle emotional stresses. It might also make her more likely to express any distress she did experience with physical rather than psychological symptoms.

Her illness first began with physical symptoms, specifically about her heart and these could be understood as a displacement of her anxiety about her mother's health. Although her urgency can be seen as a symptom of anxiety, the fact that it has become so prominent in her communication to doctors suggests that she has found it the most acceptable way to relay her distress. This pattern of 'illness behaviour' has been reinforced by her doctors dealing with her difficulties at a physical level.

It is not clear why Mrs Baker's depressive symptoms have persisted for six years. Although this could be partly due to her not having been given sufficient medication, affective disorders tend to remit spontaneously and she might have been expected to have recovered by this time. This suggests that there is likely to be some perpetuating factor. Her mother continues to have angina, but is otherwise well. Mrs Baker reports no difficulties in her marriage, apart from those she attributes to her presenting symptoms. Moreover, during the interview, her husband appears to have been an extremely supportive and non-intrusive person. Although we frequently find that a more detailed exploration of interpersonal relationships can throw light on an otherwise incomprehensible problem, there is no evidence for this at the present time.

Further investigations

At this stage it is important to obtain information from other sources. These will include records of Mrs Baker's previous contact with the gynaecologist, urologist, and psychiatrist. It would also be useful to contact her general practitioner who should be able to provide a more detailed and objective account of Mr and Mrs Baker's marriage.

Further information should also be obtained from Mrs Baker about the initial onset of her depression, how she reacted to learning about her mother's myocardial infarct, how she felt about Leonard's birth and how she responded to her own hysterectomy. Interviewing Mr and Mrs Baker together will allow a more critical evaluation to be made of the strengths and weaknesses of their marriage.

Management

The first aim will be to involve Mrs Baker and her husband in a psychological approach to her illness. This will be facilitated by a sympathetic approach and the use of psychologically-orientated questions. The foundations for establishing rapport should already have been created during the assessment interview and by encouraging Mr Baker to participate he may be able to be brought in as a therapeutic ally.

The psychiatrist will need to offer an uncomplicated and non-dogmatic explanation of Mrs Baker's symptoms, as far as he understands them, and then set out general principles for helping her. He should therefore say that he thinks she is depressed, that her depression seems to be related to the stressful events outlined above. It would then be logical for him to continue with her antidepressant and in Mrs Baker's case this would mean increasing it to a more therapeutic dose.

Treatment will include the provision of psychological support. This incorporates more detailed understanding of the nature and meaning of Mrs Baker's symptoms in the context of her personal development and her marriage.

Prognosis

The prognosis will depend upon the underlying diagnosis. Although affective disorders respond well to appropriate treatment, the long-standing nature of Mrs Baker's symptoms suggests that her recovery may not be complete. Any significant improvement will probably depend upon whether the factors that are perpetuating her symptoms can be established.

Brief formulation

Mrs Baker is a 36-year-old married woman with two children who has had an obsessional preoccupation with passing urine for the last two years. No physical cause has been found for this and it has failed to respond to previous psychiatric and surgical intervention. It has developed in the context of a six-year history of depressed mood which appears to have started soon after her son's birth, six years previously. On examination, Mrs Baker has features of a moderate depression.

Diagnosis

The most likely diagnosis is that Mrs Baker has a chronic depressive illness with obsessional features. There is no evidence to suggest that she has a physical illness.

Aetiology

Mrs Baker's depression appeared to follow soon after the birth of her second child and her mother suffering from a minor heart attack. She may have been vulnerable to these stresses because of a long-standing concern with her father's death from a heart attack, which she observed, and a considerable attachment to both her parents. Soon after the onset of this depression she had a hysterectomy, which may have contributed to the perpetuation of her symptoms. Her depression never appears to have been adequately treated but it is possible that additional fators have contributed to its perpetuation, which are not known at this stage.

Further investigations

More information is required about Mrs Baker's previous contact with doctors throughout her illness and about the state of her marriage.

Management

Mrs Baker will need psychological support and her tricyclic antidepressants should be continued in higher dosage.

Prognosis

The long-standing nature of her symptoms suggests that they will not remit completely, certainly unless any perpetuating factors have been defined and addressed.

Further information

The psychiatrist began to perceive Mrs Baker's problem as a manifestation of a depressive illness from early in the interview and he therefore started to explore this gently by the way in which he conducted his examination. By the time he completed the history and examination he felt confident that she would be able to make sense of the explanation outlined in the initial formulation.

When he conveyed this to her he observed a significant reduction in tension in both Mr and Mrs Baker who readily agreed to co-operate with his suggestions, which included increasing the dose of amitriptyline to 100 mg at night. He also advised her to

stop taking flurazepam, because of the increased sedative effect
of the tricyclic antidepressant.

The psychiatrist was also able to obtain information from the
previous doctors who had treated Mrs Baker.

The gynaecologist confirmed that he performed a hysterectomy eight months after her second child was born. No significant pathology was found and a diagnosis of dysfunctional
uterine bleeding had been made. At no time did her haemoglobin
fall below 13 g/dl.

The urologist had assessed Mrs Baker's bladder capacity both
when she had been in a conscious state as well as under general
anaesthetic. He also performed a cystoscopy. All these investigations proved normal, but he undertook a urethral dilation in the
hope that this might alleviate her symptoms.

The psychiatric report showed that her original referral was
provoked by concern that her frequency of micturition would
prevent her going on a holiday abroad with her family. She was
therefore admitted fairly urgently to hospital for treatment. A
diagnosis of an 'obsessional disorder in a person with a neurotic
personality' was made and there were frequent comments about
her 'high level of anxiety'. She was treated with a behavioural
programme, which was reported to have reduced both her level
of anxiety and her frequency of micturition sufficiently to allow
her to go on her planned holiday. The psychologist who treated
her also commented on her 'passive and inhibited nature' and
her 'difficulty in expressing negative feelings' and suggested that
marital therapy could be useful because he considered that Mr
Baker contributed to the situation by exerting too much control
over his wife.

The psychiatrist also spoke to Mr and Mrs Baker's general
practitioner, who confirmed the details of her previous treatment
including the fact that she showed moderate improvement after
her admission to the psychiatric hospital. He said that he did not
refer her back to that unit because of the incident that upset her
when she was first admitted. As far as Mr and Mrs Baker's
marriage was concerned the general practitioner said that there
were no financial problems at all, but he often wondered whether
there was any 'depth' to their relationship. He also said that her
children frequently 'take advantage of her and cause chaos'. He
agreed that he found her depressed but attributed this to her

'fixation with passing urine'. During this conversation he also informed the psychiatrist that he had restarted Mr Baker's flurazepam because she had returned to his clinic complaining of insomnia.

Two weeks later when Mrs Baker and her husband returned for their follow-up appointment they both reported a moderate, gradual improvement in her sense of well-being and in her symptoms.

Mental state examination

Appearance and behaviour

Mrs Baker looked less tense and sat in a less stiff fashion in her chair.

Talk

She was more forthcoming than previously, but continued to allow her husband to answer questions for her.

Mood

She looked much less miserable, but clearly remained unhappy. She reported an improvement in her sleeping and an increase in her appetite.

Thought content

She said she felt much more relaxed, but expressed concern that she might have made the psychiatrist cross by returning to her general practitioner for more sleeping tablets. She was now worrying about whether she was going to 'slip back' again. When she talked about her lack of self-confidence, Mrs Baker said that she was never able to do anything for herself. Even her promotion had been arranged for her by her father, who always did everything for her. She also admitted to thinking and dreaming about him much more since the last interview.

Abnormal beliefs and interpretation of events

None were elicited.

Abnormal experiences

None were elicited.

Cognitive state

Not tested.

Appraisal of illness

This was not directly discussed but Mrs Baker seemed keen to discuss her emotional problems.

The psychiatrist has acquired considerable information and should now be in a position to develop a management plan in the light of this.

Reformulation

Diagnosis

There is no change in the original diagnosis. The further information confirms that no physical explanation has been found to explain her urgency of micturition. Even her previous menorrhagia was attributed to dysfunctional uterine bleeding—a retrospective diagnosis dependent upon excluding pathology.

The first psychiatric assessment emphasized the obsessional and anxious nature of her symptoms which explains why these were specifically treated. However, these features are also consistent with a diagnosis of depression and this is further supported by her general practitioner confirming her previous mood change and her improvement following the psychiatrist's latest intervention.

Aetiology

It may be that the stresses at home are greater than Mrs Baker acknowledged during her first interview. Both her general practitioner and the psychologist she saw previously believed that her relationship with her husband was unsatisfactory because he was over-controlling. Furthermore, her children were thought difficult to control and caused her considerable problems. The fact that she appears to have no interest outside her home takes on even greater significance if her experience of family life is unsatisfactory. The psychologist also commented on her diffidence.

Although her lack of self-esteem could well be a manifestation of depression, it could also be that this is a life-long character trait which has become exaggerated by her illness.

These factors suggest ways in which Mrs Baker's relationship with her husband may have perpetuated her symptoms, particularly since she seemed to have valued her father for doing things that she felt unable to do for herself. In her marriage her husband seems to have taken on the role of organizing her life for her. She may have required this because of her lack of self-esteem, but she may also have resented it because it inhibited her wish to become independent. By nature she found it difficult to criticize people and this difficulty could have been reinforced by her husband's well-meaning motivation in trying to help. These conflicts and her long-standing difficulty in expressing them may well be contributory to her continuing depression.

Further investigations

More specific information is still required about the strengths and weaknesses in Mr and Mrs Baker's marriage. It has been suggested that Mrs Baker is undermined by her husband and her children. She also leads a very isolated existence at home and her attitude towards this might be open to change.

Treatment

Since Mrs Baker remains depressed her dose of antidepressant should be increased again until she either shows more signs of improvement or experiences side-effects. She will then need to continue on medication for at least six months after her recovery. However, the additional information obtained also suggests that there are several specific areas that could benefit from psychotherapeutic exploration and counselling.

She had several important losses which she does not appear to have mourned satisfactorily. First, there is her father's death, which has begun to occupy her thoughts again. Secondly, her hysterectomy has left her prematurely unable to have any more children. Thirdly, her mother's continuing angina threatens her with a further loss. At a suitable time it might become appropriate to encourage her to express how she feels about these situations.

Her lack of self-esteem appears to be compensated for by her husband's supportive, but possibly controlling attitude. It should be possible to undertake conjoint marital therapy, focusing on specific areas where Mrs Baker would benefit from gaining independence. As this progresses it should become clearer how the couple react to any possible change in their relationship. This reaction will provide additional information on which further strategies can be based.

Finally, Mrs Baker has already shown anxiety about asking her general practitioner for help. When patients are very distressed they frequently ask many people for help and then worry that everyone will get angry because their advice is being ignored. In this situation, particularly given the general practitioner's awareness of her problems, it is most important to reinforce his role in her treatment. This can be done by welcoming the use she makes of his services and maintaining clear and effective communication with him about her treatment.

Prognosis

It seems likely that Mrs Baker will improve initially, in the same way as she did when treated by the previous psychiatrist. There are also grounds for being more optimistic about the long-term prognosis. In spite of the uncertainties about their relationship, Mr Baker has returned to the out-patient department with his wife and still seems keen to co-operate with her treatment. Mrs Baker has also begun to talk more about her feelings of inadequacy than she did previously. Her general practitioner also appears to be interested and concerned in her outcome. Against this must be balanced the fact that she has been quite seriously ill for nearly six years and this may well limit the possibility for change.

As far as the marriage is concerned, there is always the possibility that opening up areas of conflict between the couple may lead to a disintegration in their relationship. If this threatens then the importance of her presenting symptoms in holding the marriage together might become clearer. On the other hand this appears to be unlikely since they both describe their relationship as having been satisfactory before Mrs Baker's illness developed.

Postscript

Mr and Mrs Baker continued to attend the out-patient department regularly on a monthly basis. Both Mrs Baker's depression and her urgency of micturition gradually diminished and she was able to spend the interviews exploring the following issues.

She expressed resentment at her lack of independence and feeling tied to her house and family. She also found Frank unsupportive at home, particularly with their children and she criticized him openly for giving more time to neighbours and friends than to herself.

Initially, Mr Baker appeared to accept these criticisms stoically. Eventually however he also began to complain of how his wife's demands upon his time and attention were irritating him. When they both began to criticize each other openly they were able to discuss ways in which they could organize their time to allow both of them increasing independence.

It became apparent that Mrs Baker was particularly worried about Leonard who was very headstrong. She felt torn between encouraging his independent behaviour and worrying about whether he would come to serious harm. He apparently resembled her father in many respects and her fears reflected her previous concern for her father who had ignored his general practitioner's advice after his first heart attack. She was also reminded of her father's death when her middle-aged driving instructor, to whom she had become extremely attached, died suddenly of a coronary. This occurred about a year after she first attended the out-patients. Learning to drive was particularly important to her because of the independence she expected to gain. However, she had failed her driving test on numerous occasions and had only just begun to build up the confidence to take it again. An aunt of hers was also dying of cancer at this time and a neighbour, with whom she had struck up a friendship, had been diagnosed as having cancer of the breast.

With encouragement from the psychiatrist and supported by her husband, Mrs Baker was able to express increasingly openly how angry and frightened she felt when her own father died. He had apparently ignored the advice his general practitioner had given him following his first myocardial infarction, which was to slow down and to take life easily. She had always thought he had contributed to his early death by carrying on as normal. Not only did she appear to benefit by expressing these thoughts and feelings, but she was also reassured to learn that her father's attitude to his illness was consistent with present medical attitudes.

Soon after this she passed her driving test and also found herself a part-time job working in a local school, both of which considerably increased her self-confidence.

Mrs Baker also expressed regret at having had a hysterectomy at such an early age and began to talk about how she would have liked to have had more children. Just before treatment ended she and her husband bought a puppy.

After attending the out-patient department for 18 months Mrs Baker showed considerable signs of improvement. She was no longer depressed and her presenting symptom was a rare occurrence which she spontaneously reported as being provoked by anxiety. She and her husband were much more open and relaxed together and her increased independence was appreciated by her husband, who said he felt that he and the children were less pressurized. Three months previously she had decided that she wanted to stop taking her antidepressant medication completely and was now happy to be discharged.

13

Some concluding remarks

We hope that by now the reader will have an appreciation of how we have 'made sense' of the cases presented in this book. Our intention has been to make the process manifest by describing its operation in relation to patients rather than through formal exposition. However, it seems appropriate to conclude with some general remarks about our approach in a more theoretical way. The tenor of the book would make a detailed discussion of these out of place and our aim is not to examine them exhaustively but to do little more than list some important themes. We hope that the reader will be stimulated to consider them more deeply.

Clinical judgement

Most of the information elicited about the patients in this book has been straightforward in nature, easily communicated to others, and readily obtainable by a competent interviewer. However, it will probably have been observed that we have had difficulty in articulating some aspects of clinical experience which are of great importance. The clinician uses himself as a sensitive instrument attempting to gauge certain responses induced in him by the patient in the course of the psychiatric interview. The perception of what is significant in a particular case may not depend solely on the content of what the patient says. The way in which a remark is put, the context in which it is made, the point in the course of history-taking at which it emerges, the tone of voice accompanying it, and so on may impress themselves on the clinician as being in some way noteworthy.

We have attempted in our cases to preserve these observations, but we can understand that the reader will sometimes conclude that inferences have been drawn which go well beyond the data provided. We consider, however, that some clinical judgements cannot be arrived at simply by deduction from particular observations, but depend on experience gained from previous similar cases and, sometimes, on intuition. However, it is important to bear in mind the relatively insecure foundation on which such intuitive judgements are based. It is therefore necessary to seek further information through history-taking or by direct observation in order to support or refute them.

Selection and organization

We have already noted that relevant clinical information is selected and organized in order to arrive at a formulation of the case. The use of a pre-determined structure facilitates the acquisition of this information. What is sought and what is regarded as significant are subject to constant development or modification in the light of the most recent formulation of the case. In turn, the formulation may change as new information comes to light.

The structure serves a number of important functions. It reveals omissions and areas of ignorance; it guides the clinician towards areas for further inquiry or observation; as the formulation develops, management plans suggest themselves together with their goals and means by which their effectiveness may be monitored. The formulation leads to the establishment of important hypotheses about the patient and his illness which can then be tested further. It is essentially an argument concerning the individual case. No doubt alternative structures can be brought forward but the one we have presented has a long tradition in British psychiatry and we hope that we have displayed its value.

It is worth considering whether the structure of the formulation presented in this book imposes a constraint or limitation on the way in which we think about our patients. Does it, for example, limit the types of information that we seek or commit us to a narrow range of possibilities in our conceptualization of the patient's problems? Does it impede the development of an original approach which might prove even more valuable? We do not discount these possibilities but we have found that the traditional formulation allows considerable flexibility. Many 'models' of mental illness can be subsumed and placed side by side within its framework—biological, psychodynamic, behavioural, family and social. Often this can be done without serious contradictions emerging because some problems will be best illuminated by adopting one view while others will be best illuminated using another. When contradictions do arise, points of incompatibility are exposed and the evidence, for the particular case, can be marshalled to help us decide which approach is most helpful. In the clinical formulation factors operating at a variety of conceptual levels, from the cultural to the biochemical, can be integrated in a manner which is difficult to achieve in formal terms.

The particular and the general

In all our cases the reader will be aware of our attention to two elements. On the one hand we have sought features which the patient has in common with others suffering from similar problems and on the other hand we have examined what is unique to the individual. We hope that we have demonstrated that in the formulation one must be mindful of both. Commonalities provide a link with a body of useful knowledge, empirically derived, concerning such matters as the general implications of a particular diagnosis or the likelihood that a particular treatment will be effective. However, the expression of a mental illness is also the product of the patient's uniqueness— his individual circumstances, his personality, and his past experiences. Our ability to establish a rapport or working relationship with the patient is influenced by our understanding of his way of seeing the world, his dispositions, and his interests. In our discussions with the patient about such matters as the nature of his problems, the treatment required, and the consequences of his illness we take cognizance of the 'language' he understands. Throughout the formulation, the general and the particular stand side by side, each placing in perspective the other.

Types of 'understanding'

The term 'making sense' in the title of this book is a complex one. The reader may have discerned a number of types or levels of 'understanding' which have been employed. We have already referred to the manner in which a number of 'models' of mental illness and its causation may help us to understand various aspects of the patient's problems and to devise treatment plans in accordance with their principles. In addition we should like to draw attention to another facet of 'understanding' which arises out of the clinical method described in this book.

In the aetiological formulation we have attempted to built up a picture of how the patient's problems have evolved, paying attention to his previous experiences, his vulnerabilities and resources, and his current life circumstances. These features are particular to the case and the processes involved cannot be expressed in terms of general laws. Individual details are necessary for the sequence of experiences to be comprehensible to the interviewer and he 'understands' how particular phenomena have arisen in an emphatic manner. This type of understanding (Jasper's '*verstehen*') is an every-day, practical one and depends on the interviewer's ability to see the imprint of a coherent individual consciousness or character in the patient's experiences and behaviour. We hope that the reader has been able to join us in making sense of many experiences and behaviours of the patients presented in this book in such a manner. However, it will be evident that in many instances this kind of understanding is insufficient to take us to the core of morbid phenomena to which our patients have been subject. A limit is reached beyond which the patient's experience and behaviour cannot be made sense of in this way. We might understand, for example, why the patient has become distressed given his personality and his life situation, but we cannot understand in the same sense why his illness has taken the form of a depressive psychosis rather than an anxiety state, or anorexia nervosa rather than an obsessive–compulsive neurosis. At this point we seek after a different kind of 'understanding' based on 'explanations'. Mental illnesses take the form of discontinuities in an individual's development which can be understood as catastrophes with a cause.

In contrast to emphatic 'understanding', 'causal explanations' are stated in scientific terms and are believed to follow general laws like those characterizing the natural sciences. They deal with factors, generally biological ones, operating at an extra-conscious level which can be studied using experimental methods. Their status as knowledge is different from that achieved through emphatic 'understanding'.

The formulation, as presented in this book, heeds both 'understanding' and 'explanation', 'reasons', and 'causes', and serves to define the relationships between them. Both are necessary for a full account of the development of the patient's illness.

Eclecticism in treatment

The treatment offered to the patient arises out of the diagnostic and aetiological parts of the formulation. As clinicians, we are aware that our understanding of the patient cannot rest at an academic level, but must also lead to therapeutic implications. It could be argued that the major purpose of the formulation is a practical one; it helps us to help the patient. Since the diagnostic and aetiological parts of the formulation are usually multidimensional, so are the therapeutic options which develop from them. We may find, for example, that there is a biological component which needs attention (perhaps requiring medication), a psychological component (perhaps requiring the mobilization of social supports). We may see one treatment modality as being the most important for a particular case. Generally, in the practice of hospital psychiatry, a single approach would not suffice. Often the sequencing of treatment is important, for example, giving medication first to make the patient accessible to help of a psychotherapeutic kind. The formulation acts as a corrective to the slavish adherence to a single kind of treatment.

Coda

In this concluding chapter we have suggested several reasons for considering that formulating a case is more than a dry-as-dust examination exercise. The previous chapters have been step-by-step demonstrations of how we have proceeded from a mass of information about the symptoms, personal circumstances, and wishes of a patient to a plan of treatment using the formulation available to the psychiatrist and the validity of his conclusions. We have chosen cases to be as realistic as possible, and we hope that our readers could have imagined themselves to have had the responsibility for managing them.

When comparing their formulations with ours, we shall not be surprised if some readers disagreed with us—psychiatry is, after all, not yet a very exact science, and, although we have taken pains to describe what we think is good management, there may be some courses of action which we did not consider. Whether readers agree or disagree, we shall be satisfied if they are stimulated to be more precise or more comprehensive in their formulations, especially if they feel, as we do, that careful formulation of one case hones up a basic technical skill which can then be exercised with greater economy of effort and to a higher standard in subsequent cases.

Index